# WHOLE BODY RESET DIET COOKBOOK

The Science-Backed Guide and Budget-friendly Recipes to Lose Weight and Boost Your Metabolism | For All Ages & Full Color Pictures included

**TIMOTHY A. GWIN**

# Copyright Page

# TABLE OF CONTENTS

# INTRODUCTION

Welcome to "The Whole Body Reset Diet Cookbook," where we blend the art of culinary excellence with the science of holistic wellness. In a world increasingly saturated with fast foods, processed meals, and dietary misinformation, the quest for true health and vitality can often feel overwhelming. This cookbook is not just a collection of recipes; it is a comprehensive guide designed to reset your body, reinvigorate your spirit, and realign your approach to food and wellness.

### The Philosophy Behind Whole Body Reset

The philosophy behind the Whole Body Reset is rooted in a holistic understanding of health, one that recognizes the intricate connections between diet, lifestyle, and overall well-being. Unlike conventional diets that focus solely on weight loss or calorie counting, the Whole Body Reset emphasizes nourishment, balance, and sustainability.

- **Holistic Health:** The Whole Body Reset is built on the principle that true health encompasses more than just physical fitness. It integrates mental clarity, emotional stability, and spiritual fulfillment. By focusing on nutrient-dense foods and mindful eating practices, this approach aims to harmonize the body, mind, and spirit.

- **Nutrient-Dense Foods:** At the core of the Whole Body Reset is the emphasis on nutrient-dense, whole foods. These are foods that are minimally processed and packed with vitamins, minerals, antioxidants, and other essential nutrients.

- **Mindful Eating:** Mindful eating is a cornerstone of the Whole Body Reset philosophy. It involves paying full attention to the experience of eating and drinking, both inside and outside the body.

- **Sustainability**: The Whole Body Reset is not a quick fix but a sustainable lifestyle change. It encourages habits and practices that can be maintained long-term, ensuring that the benefits you gain are lasting. This includes adopting a diet that is not only beneficial for your health but also environmentally conscious.

- **Personalization**: Recognizing that each individual is unique, the Whole Body Reset encourages personalization. It provides guidelines and principles that can be tailored to fit your specific needs, preferences, and health goals.

## HOW THIS COOKBOOK CAN TRANSFORM YOUR LIFE

The "Whole Body Reset Diet Cookbook" is designed to be more than a culinary guide; it is a transformative tool that can change the way you think about food and health. Here's how:

- **Education and Empowerment:** This cookbook empowers you with knowledge about the nutritional value of different foods, the benefits of various cooking methods, and the impact of your dietary choices on your overall health. By understanding the "why" behind the recipes, you are more likely to make informed and healthful choices.

- **Practical and Delicious Recipes:** Featuring a wide range of recipes that are both nutritious and delicious, the cookbook proves that healthy eating does not have to be boring or restrictive. It includes meals for all times of the day, catering to different tastes and dietary requirements, ensuring that everyone can find something they love.

- **Step-by-Step Guidance:** Each recipe is accompanied by step-by-step instructions, making it easy for even novice cooks to prepare wholesome meals. The cookbook also includes tips on meal planning, grocery shopping, and efficient cooking techniques, helping you to integrate healthy eating into your daily routine seamlessly.

- **Balanced Meal Plans:** The cookbook offers sample meal plans that are balanced and designed to meet various health goals, whether you are looking to lose weight, build muscle, boost energy, or improve digestion. These meal plans take the guesswork out of what to eat and ensure you are getting a variety of nutrients.

# UNDERSTANDING YOUR BODY

The human body is a complex and highly organized structure, composed of various systems that work in concert to maintain homeostasis and support life. It can be divided into several levels of structural organization, from the smallest chemical level to the largest organismal level.

- **Cellular Level:** Cells are the basic units of life. The human body is composed of trillions of cells, each performing specific functions necessary for survival.
- **Tissue Level:** Tissues are groups of similar cells that perform a common function. There are four basic types of tissues: epithelial, connective, muscle, and nervous tissue.
- **Organ Level:** Organs are structures composed of at least two types of tissues that work together to perform specific functions. Examples include the heart, liver, and lungs.
- **Organ System Level:** Organ systems consist of related organs that work together to achieve a common purpose. The human body has eleven major organ systems, including the circulatory, respiratory, digestive, and nervous systems.
- **Organismal Level:** The organismal level is the highest level of organization, representing the sum total of all structural levels working in unison to support life.

**Key Organ Systems**

- Circulatory System: Composed of the heart, blood vessels, and blood, this system transports oxygen, nutrients, and hormones to cells and removes waste products.
- Respiratory System: Includes the lungs and airways, facilitating the exchange of oxygen and carbon dioxide.
- Digestive System: Involves organs such as the stomach, intestines, and liver, which work together to break down food and absorb nutrients.
- Nervous System: Consists of the brain, spinal cord, and peripheral nerves, controlling and coordinating body activities.
- Musculoskeletal System: Comprises bones, muscles, and connective tissues, providing structure and enabling movement.

## THE SCIENCE OF METABOLISM

Metabolism encompasses all chemical reactions that occur within the body to maintain life. It involves two fundamental processes:

- **Catabolism:** The breakdown of complex molecules into simpler ones, releasing energy. This includes the digestion of food and the breakdown of glucose during cellular respiration.
- **Anabolism:** The synthesis of complex molecules from simpler ones, requiring energy. This process includes the formation of proteins from amino acids and the synthesis of nucleic acids.

# METABOLIC PATHWAYS

- **Glycolysis:** The process of breaking down glucose to pyruvate, producing ATP and NADH. It occurs in the cytoplasm of cells and does not require oxygen.
- **Citric Acid Cycle (Krebs Cycle):** A series of reactions occurring in the mitochondria, producing ATP, NADH, and FADH2 from the oxidation of acetyl-CoA.
- **Oxidative Phosphorylation:** The process of ATP production in the mitochondria, driven by the transfer of electrons through the electron transport chain and the resulting proton gradient.

# FACTORS AFFECTING METABOLISM

- **Genetics**: Individual genetic makeup can influence metabolic rate and efficiency.
- **Age**: Metabolic rate generally decreases with age due to loss of muscle mass and hormonal changes.
- **Sex**: Males typically have a higher metabolic rate than females due to greater muscle mass.
- **Hormones**: Hormones such as thyroxine, insulin, and adrenaline play significant roles in regulating metabolism.
- **Physical Activity**: Exercise increases metabolic rate by building muscle mass and enhancing energy expenditure.

# NUTRITIONAL BUILDING BLOCKS FOR A HEALTHY BODY

Proper nutrition is essential for maintaining overall health and supporting bodily functions. The body requires a balance of macronutrients, micronutrients, and water.

## Macronutrients

- **Carbohydrates:** The primary source of energy, found in foods such as grains, fruits, and vegetables. Carbohydrates are broken down into glucose, which fuels cellular activities.
- **Proteins:** Essential for growth, repair, and maintenance of tissues. Proteins are composed of amino acids, which are the building blocks for enzymes, hormones, and structural components of the body. Sources include meat, fish, eggs, dairy, legumes, and nuts.
- **Fats:** Necessary for energy storage, cell membrane structure, and hormone production. Healthy fats include unsaturated fats from sources like olive oil, avocados, and nuts. Saturated fats and trans fats, found in processed foods, should be limited.

## Micronutrients

**Vitamins:** Organic compounds required in small quantities for various bodily functions. Key vitamins include:

- Vitamin A: Important for vision, immune function, and skin health.
- Vitamin C: Necessary for collagen synthesis, antioxidant protection, and immune support.
- Vitamin D: Crucial for calcium absorption and bone health.
- Vitamin E: An antioxidant that protects cells from damage.
- Vitamin K: Essential for blood clotting and bone health.

**Minerals:** Inorganic elements required for various physiological functions. Key minerals include:

- Calcium: Important for bone and teeth health, muscle function, and nerve signaling.
- Iron: Essential for the formation of hemoglobin, which carries oxygen in the blood.
- Magnesium: Involved in over 300 biochemical reactions, including energy production and muscle function.
- Potassium: Crucial for maintaining fluid balance, nerve transmission, and muscle contractions.

## Water

Water is vital for life, accounting for about 60% of body weight. It is involved in numerous bodily functions, including:

- Temperature Regulation: Through sweating and respiration.
- Nutrient Transport: As a solvent for nutrients and minerals.
- Waste Removal: Via urine and feces.
- Lubrication and Cushioning: For joints and tissues.

## Maintaining a Healthy Metabolism and Body

- Balanced Diet: Consuming a variety of foods to ensure adequate intake of all essential nutrients.
- Regular Exercise: Engaging in both aerobic and resistance training to boost metabolic rate and maintain muscle mass.
- Hydration: Drinking sufficient water to support metabolic processes and overall health.

- Adequate Sleep: Ensuring restful sleep to allow for recovery and hormonal balance.
- Stress Management: Utilizing techniques such as meditation, yoga, or deep breathing to reduce the negative impact of stress on metabolism.

# FUNDAMENTALS OF THE WHOLE BODY RESET DIET

The Whole Body Reset Diet is a comprehensive nutritional approach designed to rejuvenate the body, improve metabolic health, and support sustainable weight management. This diet emphasizes whole, nutrient-dense foods while avoiding processed and inflammatory ingredients. Let's delve into its core principles and outline the foods to embrace and avoid for optimal health benefits.

## CORE PRINCIPLES

**Nutrient Density Over Caloric Restriction:**

- The Whole Body Reset Diet prioritizes foods rich in vitamins, minerals, antioxidants, and other essential nutrients. Instead of focusing on calorie counting, this diet encourages the consumption of nutrient-dense foods that provide the body with the essential compounds it needs to function optimally.

**Whole Foods Focus:**

- Emphasis is placed on whole, unprocessed foods. This includes fresh fruits, vegetables, whole grains, lean proteins, and healthy fats. By minimizing processed foods, the diet aims to reduce the intake of artificial additives, preservatives, and other potentially harmful substances.

**Balanced Macronutrient Intake:**

- The diet ensures a balanced intake of carbohydrates, proteins, and fats. This balance helps stabilize blood sugar levels, reduce cravings, and support overall metabolic health.

**Anti-Inflammatory Approach:**

- Reducing inflammation is a key aspect of the Whole Body Reset Diet. Chronic inflammation is linked to numerous health issues, including obesity, diabetes, and cardiovascular diseases.

**Hydration:**

- Adequate hydration is vital for all bodily functions. The diet encourages regular water intake and the consumption of hydrating foods, such as fruits and vegetables with high water content.

**Mindful Eating:**

- Mindful eating practices are integral to the diet. This involves paying attention to hunger and fullness cues, eating slowly, and savoring each bite.

**Personalization and Flexibility:**

- Recognizing that each individual has unique dietary needs and preferences, the Whole Body Reset Diet allows for personalization. It provides guidelines but encourages individuals to tailor the diet to their specific health goals and lifestyle.

# FOODS TO EMBRACE

**Vegetables:**

- Cruciferous vegetables (broccoli, cauliflower, Brussels sprouts)
- Leafy greens (spinach, kale, Swiss chard)
- Root vegetables (sweet potatoes, carrots, beets)
- Other vegetables (bell peppers, zucchini, cucumbers)

**Fruits:**

- Berries (blueberries, strawberries, raspberries)
- Citrus fruits (oranges, grapefruits, lemons)
- Apples, pears, bananas, and other seasonal fruits

**Whole Grains:**

- Quinoa, brown rice, oats, barley, and whole wheat products
- Ancient grains like farro, spelt, and millet

**Lean Proteins:**

- Poultry (chicken, turkey)
- Fish and seafood (salmon, mackerel, sardines)
- Plant-based proteins (beans, lentils, chickpeas, tofu, tempeh)
- Lean cuts of meat (beef, pork)

**Healthy Fats:**

- Nuts and seeds (almonds, walnuts, chia seeds, flaxseeds)
- Avocados
- Olive oil, coconut oil, and other unrefined plant oils

**Dairy and Dairy Alternatives:**

- Low-fat or fat-free dairy (yogurt, milk, cheese)
- Fortified plant-based milk (almond milk, soy milk, oat milk)

**Herbs and Spices:**

- Fresh herbs (basil, cilantro, parsley)
- Spices (turmeric, ginger, cinnamon, garlic)

# FOODS TO AVOID

**Processed Foods:**

- Packaged snacks (chips, cookies, crackers)
- Processed meats (sausages, hot dogs, deli meats)
- Pre-made meals (frozen dinners, boxed meals)

**Refined Carbohydrates:**

- White bread, white pasta, and white rice
- Pastries, cakes, and sweets made with refined flour

**Sugary Foods and Beverages:**

- Sodas and sugary drinks (including fruit juices with added sugars)
- Candy, chocolates, and desserts with high sugar content
- Sweetened breakfast cereals and granola bars

**Unhealthy Fats:**

- Trans fats (found in many fried foods and commercially baked goods)
- Hydrogenated oils and partially hydrogenated oils
- Excessive amounts of saturated fats (from sources like butter, lard, and fatty cuts of meat)

**Artificial Additives:**

- Artificial sweeteners (aspartame, sucralose)
- Preservatives and artificial colorings
- Flavor enhancers like monosodium glutamate (MSG)

**High-Sodium Foods:**

- Processed and canned soups
- Salty snacks (pretzels, salted nuts)
- High-sodium condiments (soy sauce, certain salad dressings)

**Alcohol and Caffeine:**

- Limit alcohol consumption
- Moderate caffeine intake, particularly avoiding sugary caffeinated drinks

## IMPLEMENTING THE WHOLE BODY RESET DIET

To successfully implement the Whole Body Reset Diet, start by gradually incorporating more whole foods into your meals and phasing out processed items. Planning and preparing meals ahead of time can help ensure you have nutritious options available, reducing the temptation to opt for less healthy choices. It's also beneficial to keep a food journal to track your progress and observe how different foods affect your body and mood.

Engaging in regular physical activity, managing stress through practices like meditation or yoga, and ensuring adequate sleep are also critical components that complement the dietary guidelines of the Whole Body Reset Diet.

# SETTING UP YOUR KITCHEN FOR SUCCESS

Setting up your kitchen effectively is a crucial step toward achieving culinary success and maintaining a healthy lifestyle. A well-organized kitchen not only enhances efficiency but also inspires creativity and reduces stress during meal preparation. This comprehensive guide will walk you through the essential steps to set up your kitchen, covering everything from organizing your space to selecting the right tools and appliances.

## ORGANIZING YOUR KITCHEN SPACE

### Assessing Your Kitchen Layout

- Understanding Your Work Triangle: The work triangle concept connects the sink, stove, and refrigerator, forming a triangular workflow. This layout minimizes movement and maximizes efficiency.
- Zoning Your Kitchen: Divide your kitchen into zones such as preparation, cooking, cleaning, and storage. Each zone should have everything you need for specific tasks, reducing the need to move back and forth.

### Decluttering and Maximizing Storage

- Declutter Your Space: Start by removing items you rarely use. Donate or discard duplicates and non-essential gadgets.
- Maximize Vertical Space: Use wall-mounted shelves, pegboards, and hooks to keep frequently used tools within reach.

- Utilize Cabinet Organizers: Incorporate pull-out shelves, drawer dividers, and lazy Susans to make the most of your cabinet space.
- Clear Countertops: Keep countertops as clear as possible to provide ample workspace for meal preparation.

## ESSENTIAL KITCHEN TOOLS AND EQUIPMENT

### Basic Tools for Every Kitchen

- **Chef's Knife**: A versatile, sharp knife is indispensable for chopping, slicing, and dicing.
- **Cutting Board**: Invest in a durable, easy-to-clean cutting board, preferably one for meat and another for vegetables to prevent cross-contamination.
- **Measuring Cups and Spoons**: Accurate measurements are key to successful recipes.
- **Mixing Bowls**: Have a set of mixing bowls in various sizes for different tasks.
- **Pots and Pans**: Essential cookware includes a sauté pan, a saucepan, and a stockpot.
- **Baking Sheets and Pans**: Necessary for baking and roasting.
- **Utensils**: Tongs, spatulas, whisks, ladles, and wooden spoons should be within easy reach.

### Small Appliances

- **Blender or Food Processor**: Great for smoothies, soups, and sauces.
- **Microwave**: Useful for quick reheating and defrosting.
- **Toaster or Toaster Oven**: For toasting and small baking tasks.

# WHITE BREAKFAST SMOOTHIE

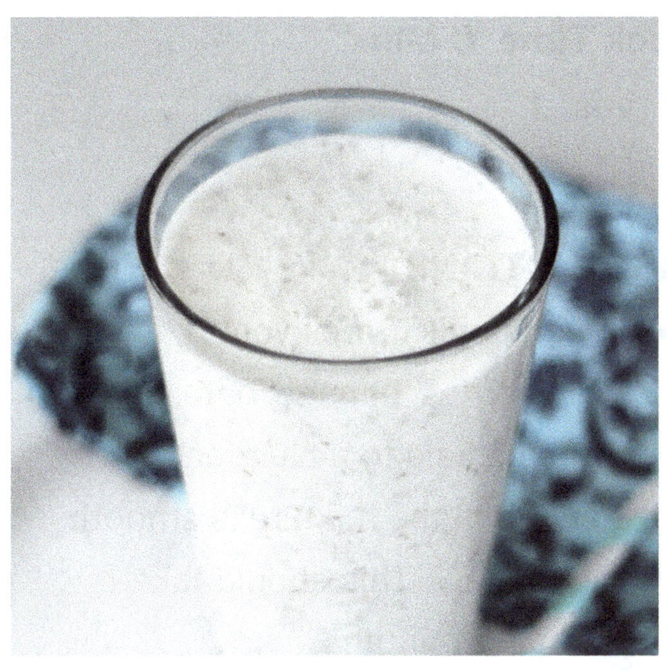

**Cook Time: 0 Mins**

**Serves: 1**

## INSTRUCTIONS

- Combine all the ingredients in a blender.
- Blend on high until the mixture is smooth, which should take about 1-2 minutes.
- Pour the smoothie into a glass and top with a pinch of cinnamon before serving.

## INGREDIENTS

- 1 small banana
- 1 red apple, cored and chopped
- 1/2 cup plain Greek yogurt
- 1/4 cup raw almonds
- 1 cup nonfat milk
- A pinch of cinnamon

## NUTRITIONAL FACTS

- Calories: 350kcal
- Protein: 20g
- Fiber: 5g
- Fat: 10g
- Sugar: 30g

# KALE AND HEARTY SMOOTHIE

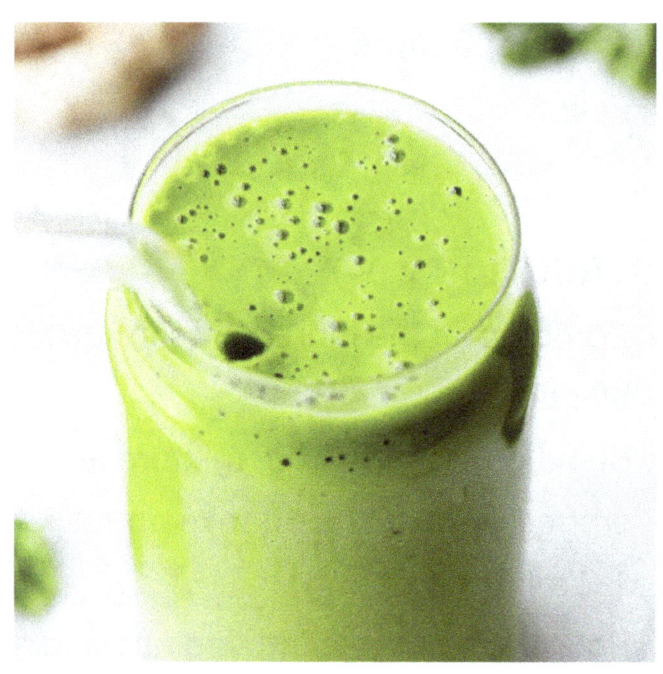

**Cook Time: 0 Mins**

**Serves: 1**

## INSTRUCTIONS

- Add the milk, Greek yogurt, frozen strawberries, banana, oats, and chopped kale to a blender.
- Blend until the mixture is smooth and creamy. This should take about 1-2 minutes.

## INGREDIENTS

- 1 cup of 1% milk
- ½ cup of plain low-fat Greek yogurt
- 1 cup of frozen strawberries
- ½ of a small banana
- ⅓ cup of oats
- ½ cup of fresh, chopped kale

## NUTRITIONAL FACTS

- Protein: 25g
- Fiber: 7g
- Calories: 374kcal

# OATMEAL WITH BERRIES AND NUTS

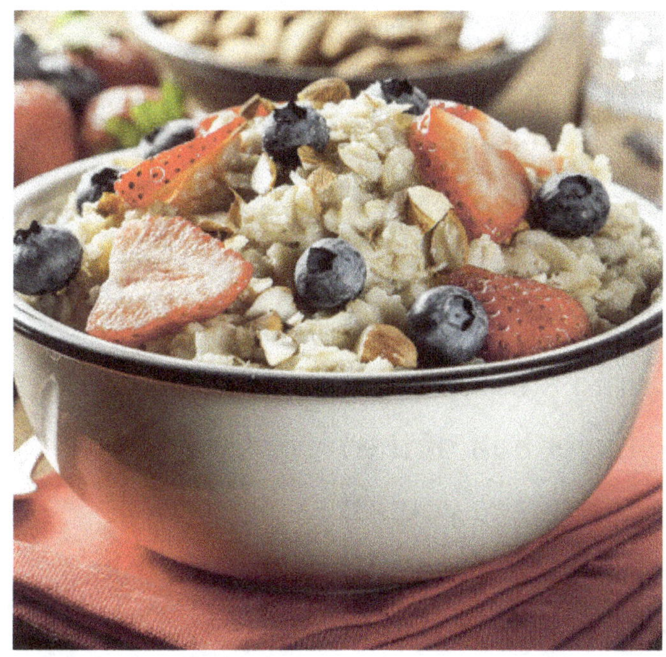

## INGREDIENTS

- 1/2 cup rolled oats
- 1 cup water or milk (for a creamier consistency)
- 1/4 cup fresh or frozen berries (e.g., blueberries, strawberries, raspberries)
- 2 tablespoons chopped nuts (such as walnuts, almonds, pecans, or cashews)
- 1 teaspoon honey or maple syrup (optional)
- 1/4 teaspoon ground cinnamon (optional)

**Cook Time: 7 Mins**

**Serves: 1**

## INSTRUCTIONS

- In a small saucepan, combine the oats and water or milk.
- Bring the mixture to a boil over high heat, then reduce the heat to low.
- Let it simmer for about 5 minutes, or until the oats are fully cooked.
- Stir in the berries, nuts, and, if desired, the honey or maple syrup and cinnamon.
- Serve warm and enjoy!

## NUTRITIONAL FACTS

- Calories: 400kcal (depending on milk choice and use of sweeteners)
- Protein: 15g
- Fiber: 7g

# GREEK YOGURT PARFAIT

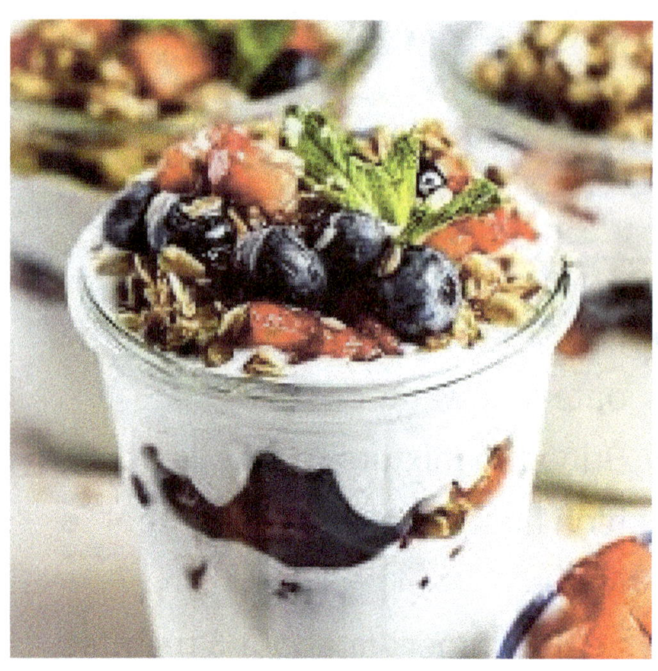

**Prep Time: 5 Mins**

**Serves: 1**

## INGREDIENTS

- 1 cup plain Greek yogurt
- 1/2 cup mixed berries (such as strawberries, blueberries, and raspberries)
- 1/4 cup granola
- Honey or maple syrup, to taste (optional)
- Ground cinnamon, to taste (optional)
- Fresh mint leaves for garnish (optional)

## INSTRUCTIONS

- Spoon half of the Greek yogurt into a serving glass or bowl.
- Layer half of the mixed berries on top of the yogurt.
- Sprinkle with half of the granola.
- Repeat the process with the remaining yogurt, berries, and granola.
- Add a drizzle of honey or maple syrup and a sprinkle of ground cinnamon, if desired.
- Garnish with fresh mint leaves for a refreshing touch.

## NUTRITIONAL FACTS

- Calories: 290-350kcal (depending on the addition of honey or syrup)
- Protein: 20g
- Fiber: 3g

# SPINACH AND MUSHROOM OMELETTE

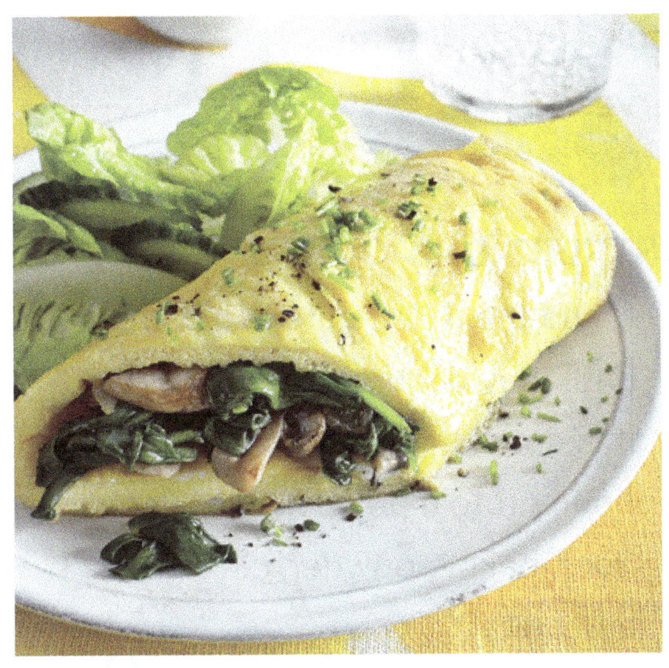



## INGREDIENTS

- 2 teaspoons extra virgin olive oil
- 2 cups sliced mushrooms
- 1 chopped onion
- 4 cups spinach, stems removed if necessary
- 4 eggs, whisked
- Salt and pepper, to taste
- 1 teaspoon dried oregano

## NUTRITIONAL FACTS

- Calories: 221 kcal
- Carbohydrates: 12g
- Protein: 16g
- Fat: 13g
- Fiber: 4g
- Sugar: 5g

## INSTRUCTIONS

- Heat 1 teaspoon of olive oil in a non-stick skillet over medium heat.
- Add the mushrooms and onions to the pan. Cook for 3 minutes, then add the spinach.
- Season the vegetables with salt, pepper, and oregano. Once the vegetables reach your preferred tenderness, transfer them to a plate.
- In the same skillet, add the remaining teaspoon of olive oil and pour in the whisked eggs.
- Sprinkle the eggs with a bit more oregano, salt, and pepper.
- Once the eggs begin to set, place the cooked vegetables on one side of the omelette.
- Use a spatula to fold the omelette in half over the vegetables.
- Cooking until the eggs are fully set and cooked to your liking.

# PROTEIN PANCAKES

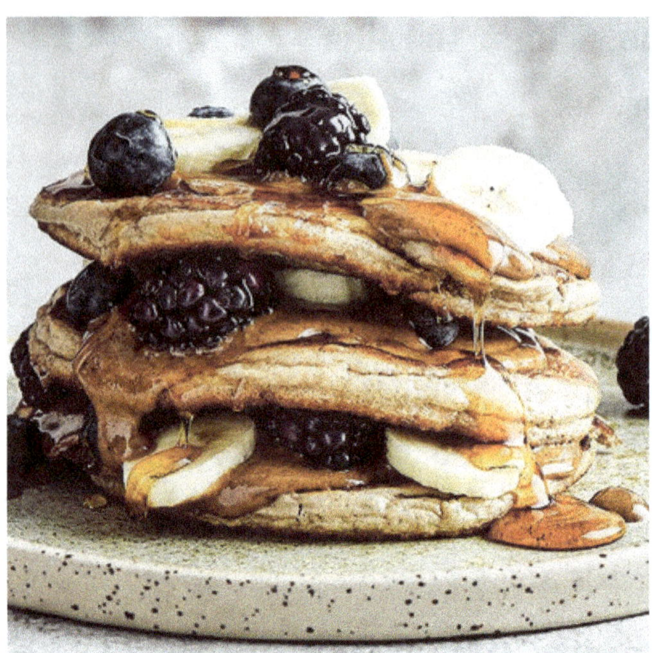

**Cook Time: 10 Mins**

**Serves: 2**

## INGREDIENTS

- 1/2 cup rolled oats
- 1 scoop of protein powder (whey or plant-based)
- 1 medium banana
- 1 large egg
- 1/4 cup milk (dairy or plant-based)
- 1 tablespoon coconut flour
- 1/2 teaspoon cinnamon
- 1 teaspoon baking powder
- Pinch of salt
- Oil, butter, or ghee for cooking

## NUTRITIONAL FACTS

Calories: 450 kcal | Fiber: 5g | Fat: 10g

Protein: 37g | Carbohydrates: 40g

## INSTRUCTIONS

- Blend the rolled oats in a blender until they become a fine flour.
- In a small bowl, combine the oat flour, protein powder, coconut flour, baking powder, cinnamon, and salt.
- In another bowl, mash the banana, then whisk in the egg and milk until the mixture is smooth.
- Add the wet mixture to the dry ingredients and stir until just combined.
- Heat a non-stick skillet over medium heat and lightly grease with oil, butter, or ghee. Pour the batter into the skillet to form pancakes. Cook until bubbles appear on the surface, then flip and cook until the pancakes are golden brown on both sides.

# CHIA SEED PUDDING RECIPE

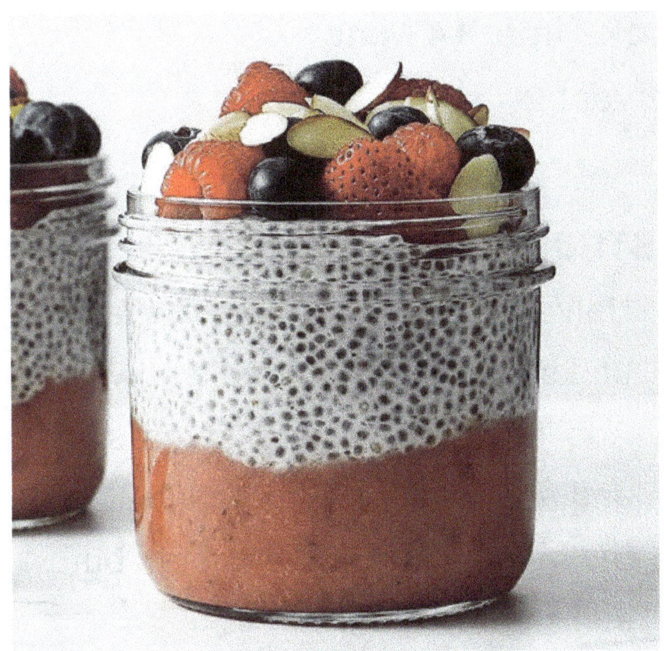

**Refrigerate Time: 4 Hours**

**Serves: 2**

## INSTRUCTIONS

- Combine chia seeds and milk: In a bowl or a mason jar, mix the chia seeds with the almond milk.
- Add sweetness and flavor: Stir in the vanilla extract and maple syrup.
- Refrigerate: Cover the mixture and place it in the refrigerator for at least 4 hours, or overnight, until it reaches a pudding-like consistency.
- Serve with toppings: Just before serving, garnish with fresh fruits of your choice.

## INGREDIENTS

- 1/4 cup chia seeds
- 1 cup unsweetened almond milk (or any plant-based milk of your choice)
- 1/2 teaspoon vanilla extract
- 1 tablespoon maple syrup (or your preferred sweetener)
- Fresh fruits for topping (e.g., berries, sliced banana)

## NUTRITIONAL FACTS

- Calories: 200 kcal
- Protein: 5g
- Carbohydrates: 20g
- Fiber: 15g
- Fat: 10g

# AVOCADO TOAST WITH POACHED EGG

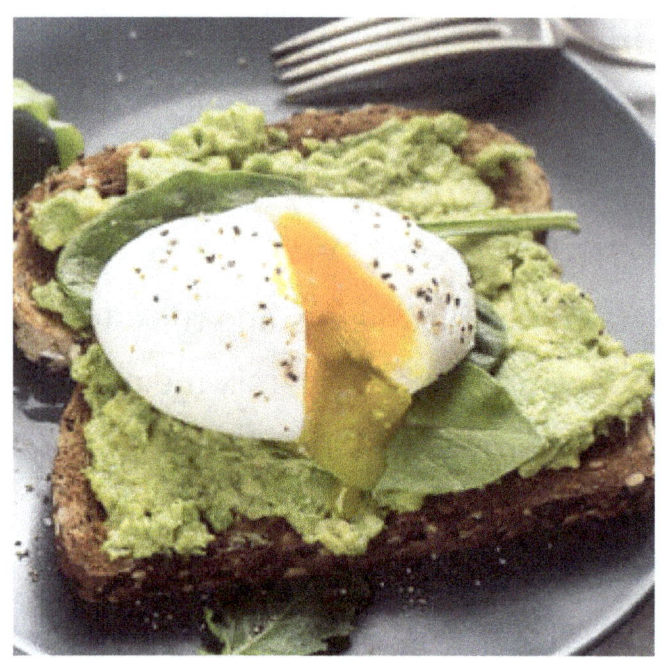

**Cook Time: 14 Mins**

**Serves: 2**

## INGREDIENTS

- 2 large eggs
- 2 slices of whole-grain bread
- 1 ripe avocado
- 1 small garlic clove, minced
- Juice of 1/2 a lime
- Pinch of salt
- Pinch of red pepper flakes (optional)
- Sprinkle of 'Everything but the Bagel' seasoning (optional)

## NUTRITIONAL FACTS

Calories: 306 kcal | Fat: 20g

Protein: 11g | Carbs: 24g

Fiber: 7g | Sugar: 2g

## INSTRUCTIONS

- Halve the avocado, remove the pit, and scoop the flesh into a bowl. Add lime juice, minced garlic, salt, and red pepper flakes. Mash until the mixture is mostly smooth but still slightly chunky.
- Fill a pot with water and bring it to a gentle boil. Crack each egg into a small cup and gently slide it into the water. Cook for about 4 minutes for a soft yolk or longer if you prefer a firmer yolk.
- While the eggs are cooking, toast the bread slices until they reach your desired level of crispiness.
- Spread the mashed avoca
- do evenly on each slice of toasted bread. Carefully remove the poached eggs from the water with a slotted spoon, drain on a paper towel, and place one egg on each slice of avocado toast.
- Sprinkle and serve immediately.

# SWEET POTATO HASH

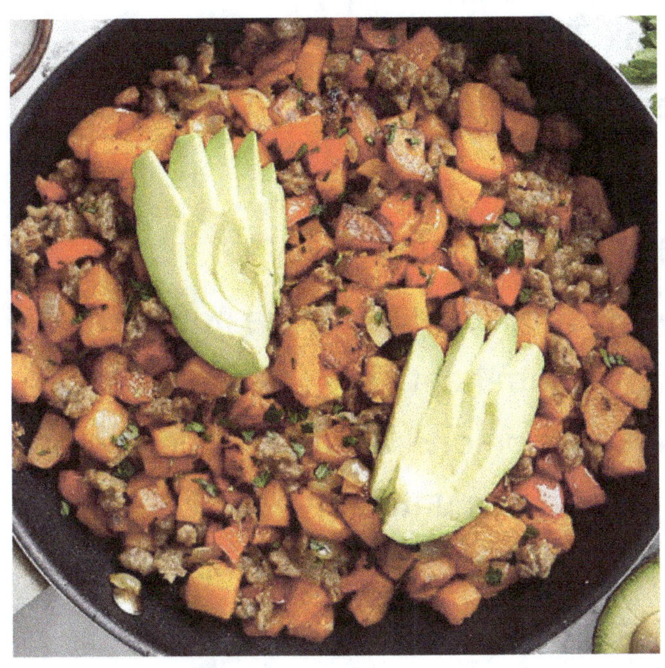

**Cook Time: 24 Mins**

**Serves: 3**

## INGREDIENTS

- 2 medium sweet potatoes, peeled and diced
- 1 tablespoon olive oil
- 1/2 red onion, diced
- 1 red bell pepper, diced
- 2 cloves garlic, minced
- Salt and pepper to taste
- Fresh parsley, chopped (for garnish)

## NUTRITIONAL FACTS

- Calories: 200kcal
- Protein: 3g
- Carbohydrates: 38g
- Fiber: 6g
- Fat: 4g

## INSTRUCTIONS

- Place the diced sweet potatoes in a microwave-safe bowl. Microwave for 3 minutes to soften them.
- In a large skillet, heat the olive oil over medium heat. Add the softened sweet potatoes and cook for about 5 minutes until they start to brown.
- Stir in the diced onion and minced garlic. Continue cooking for 3 minutes, or until the onion becomes translucent.
- Mix in the diced red bell pepper and cook for another 3 minutes.
- Season with salt and pepper to taste. Garnish with chopped fresh parsley. Serve hot.

# LENTIL SOUP

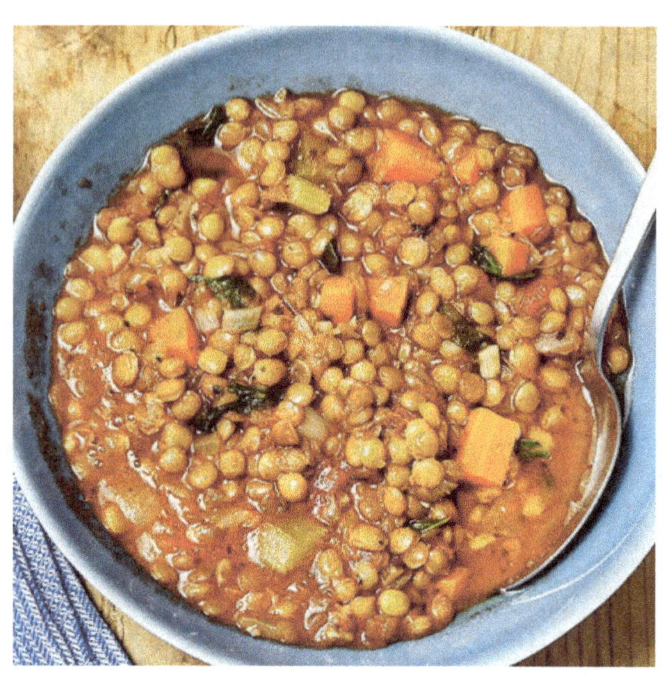

**Cook Time: 45 Mins**

**Serves: 4**

## INGREDIENTS

- 1 cup dried green or brown lentils, rinsed
- 1 large onion, diced
- 2 carrots, peeled and diced
- 2 celery stalks, diced
- 3 garlic cloves, minced
- 1 teaspoon ground cumin
- 1/2 teaspoon ground coriander
- 1/2 teaspoon smoked paprika
- 1 bay leaf
- 1 can (14 oz) diced tomatoes
- 6 cups vegetable broth
- 2 cups spinach, roughly chopped
- 1 lemon, zest and juice
- Salt and pepper, to taste
- 2 tablespoons olive oil

## INSTRUCTIONS

- Heat olive oil in a large pot over medium heat.
- Sauté onion, carrots, and celery for 5 minutes until soft.
- Add garlic, cumin, coriander, and smoked paprika, and cook for 1 minute.
- Stir in lentils, diced tomatoes, bay leaf, and vegetable broth. Bring to a boil.
- Reduce heat, cover, and simmer for 30 minutes until lentils are tender.
- Remove bay leaf, add spinach, lemon zest, and juice. Stir until spinach wilts.
- Season with salt and pepper. Serve hot with a lemon wedge.

## NUTRITIONAL FACTS

- Calories: 250 | Protein: 18g
- Carbs: 38g | Fat: 4g
- Fiber: 15g | Sugar: 5g

# GRILLED CHICKEN SALAD

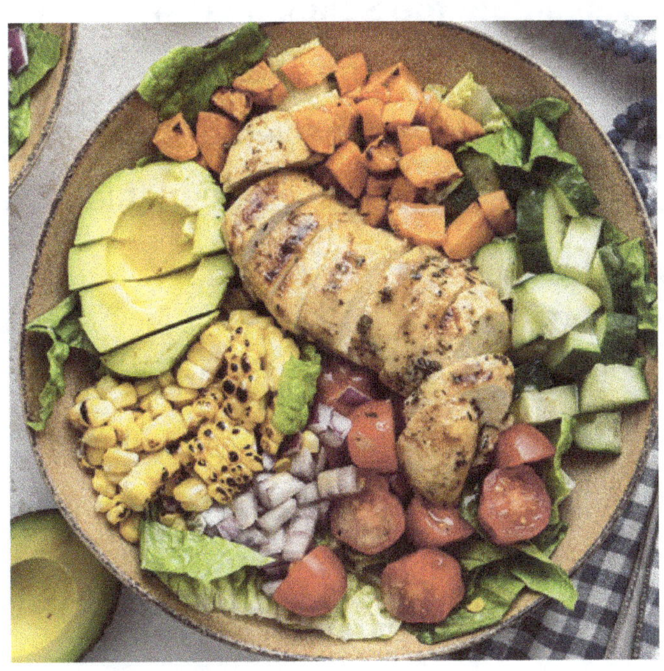

**Cook Time: 30 Mins**

**Serves: 2**

## INSTRUCTIONS

- **Prepare the Grill:** Preheat your grill to medium-high heat.
- **Marinate the Chicken:** In a bowl, mix together 1 tbsp olive oil, 1 tbsp lemon juice, 1 tsp Dijon mustard, 1 tsp honey, minced garlic, smoked paprika, onion powder, dried thyme, dried oregano, salt, and pepper. Coat the chicken breasts with this mixture and let it marinate for at least 15 minutes.
- **Grill the Chicken:** Place the marinated chicken breasts on the preheated grill. Cook for 5-7 minutes on each side, or until the internal temperature reaches 165°F (74°C). Once done, let the chicken rest for a few minutes before slicing it.

## INGREDIENTS

**For the Chicken:**

- 2 boneless, skinless chicken breasts
- 1 tbsp olive oil
- 1 tbsp lemon juice
- 1 tsp Dijon mustard
- 1 tsp honey (or sugar-free alternative)
- 1 garlic clove, minced
- 1/2 tsp smoked paprika
- 1/2 tsp onion powder
- 1/2 tsp dried thyme
- 1/2 tsp dried oregano
- Salt and pepper to taste

## INGREDIENTS

**For the Salad:**

- 4 cups chopped romaine lettuce
- 1 cup cherry tomatoes, halved
- 1 cucumber, sliced
- 1/4 red onion, thinly sliced
- 1 avocado, sliced

**For the Lemon Vinaigrette:**

- 3 tbsp olive oil
- 1 tbsp lemon juice
- 1 tsp Dijon mustard
- 1/2 tsp Italian seasoning
- 1/4 tsp garlic powder
- Salt and pepper to taste

## NUTRITIONAL FACTS

- Calories: 400kcal
- Protein: 35g
- Carbohydrates: 18g
- Fat: 22g
- Fiber: 6g
- Sugar: 5g

## INSTRUCTIONS

- **Assemble the Salad:** In a large bowl, combine the chopped romaine lettuce, halved cherry tomatoes, sliced cucumber, thinly sliced red onion, and sliced avocado.
- **Prepare the Vinaigrette:** In a small bowl, whisk together 3 tbsp olive oil, 1 tbsp lemon juice, 1 tsp Dijon mustard, Italian seasoning, garlic powder, salt, and pepper.
- **Serve:** Add the sliced grilled chicken to the salad. Drizzle with the lemon vinaigrette, toss to combine, and serve immediately.

# TURKEY AND HUMMUS WRAP

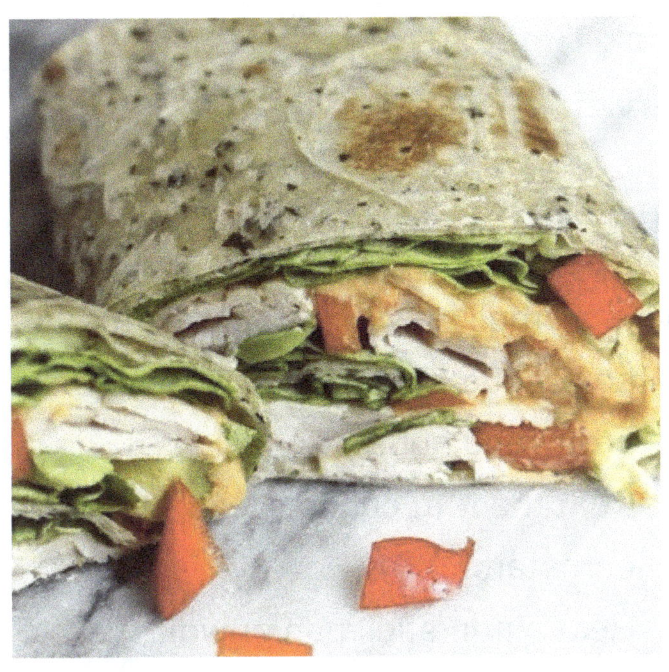

**Cook Time: 0 Mins**

**Serves: 2**

## INGREDIENTS

- 2 whole wheat tortillas (6-inch)
- 4 tablespoons hummus
- 6 ounces of sliced turkey breast (preferably free of nitrates and nitrites)
- 1/2 cup of mixed greens (such as spinach, arugula, or lettuce)
- 1/2 cucumber, thinly sliced into ribbons
- 1/2 bell pepper, cut into strips
- 1/4 red onion, thinly sliced
- Salt and pepper to taste

## INSTRUCTIONS

- Place the tortillas on a flat surface.
- Spread 2 tablespoons of hummus evenly over each tortilla.
- Layer 3 ounces of turkey slices on top of the hummus on each tortilla.
- Evenly distribute the mixed greens, cucumber ribbons, bell pepper strips, and red onion slices on the tortillas.
- Season with salt and pepper as desired.
- Roll up each tortilla tightly, tucking in the sides to secure the fillings.
- Slice each wrap in half and serve immediately.

## NUTRITIONAL FACTS

- Calories: 300kcal | Protein: 24g
- Carbohydrates: 24g | Fat: 12g
- Fiber: 5g | Sugar: 3g

# VEGETABLE STIR-FRY WITH TOFU

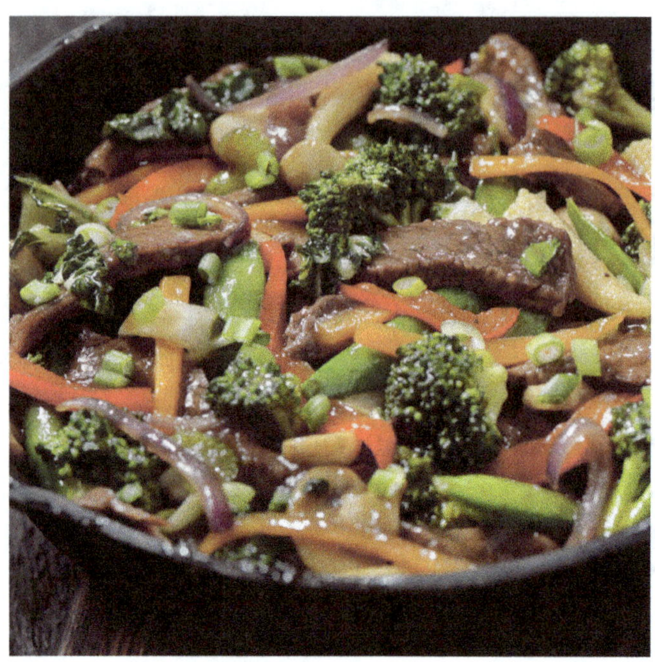

**Cook Time: 30 Mins**

**Serves: 3**

## INGREDIENTS

- 1 block of extra-firm tofu, pressed and cubed
- 2 cups of mixed vegetables (such as broccoli, bell peppers, carrots, and snap peas)
- 2 tablespoons soy sauce (or tamari for a gluten-free option)
- 1 tablespoon sesame oil
- 1 tablespoon vegetable broth
- 1 teaspoon honey (or maple syrup for a vegan option)
- 2 cloves garlic, minced
- 1 inch fresh ginger, grated
- 1 tablespoon cornstarch
- Salt to taste (optional)

## INSTRUCTIONS

- In a small bowl, mix together the soy sauce, sesame oil, vegetable broth, and honey. Set aside.
- Coat the tofu cubes evenly with cornstarch.
- Heat a non-stick pan or wok over medium-high heat. Add the tofu and cook until all sides are golden brown, about 5 minutes. Remove the tofu and set aside.
- In the same pan, add more sesame oil if necessary and sauté the garlic and ginger until aromatic.
- Add the mixed vegetables and stir-fry until they are tender but still crisp.
- Return the tofu to the pan. Pour the sauce over the tofu and vegetables, stirring to combine. Cook for another 2-3 minutes.
- Serve hot, garnished with sesame seeds or green onions if desired

# BAKED SALMON WITH STEAMED BROCCOLI

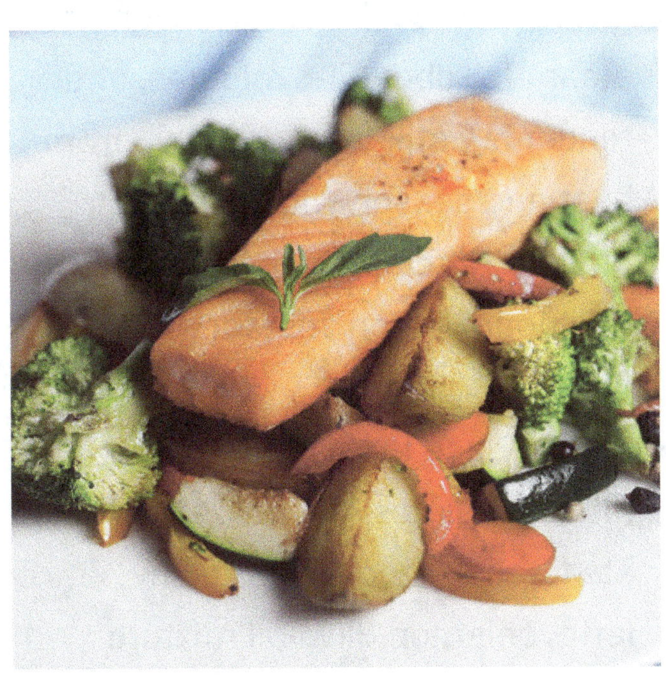

**Cook Time: 20 Mins**

**Serves: 4**

## INGREDIENTS

- 4 salmon fillets (approximately 6 ounces each)
- 2 tablespoons olive oil
- 2 garlic cloves, minced
- Juice and zest of 1 lemon
- 1 teaspoon dried dill or fresh dill to taste
- Salt and freshly ground black pepper, to taste
- 1 large head of broccoli, cut into florets
- Optional: a pinch of red pepper flakes or extra lemon zest for garnish

## INSTRUCTIONS

- Set your oven to 400°F (200°C). Prepare a baking sheet by lining it with parchment paper or lightly greasing it with olive oil.
- In a small bowl, combine olive oil, minced garlic, lemon juice and zest, dill, salt, and pepper. Place the salmon fillets on the prepared baking sheet and brush them with the mixture.
- Bake the Salmon: Bake the salmon in the preheated oven for 12-15 minutes, or until it flakes easily with a fork. Cooking time may vary based on the thickness of the fillets.
- Steam the Broccoli: While the salmon is baking, bring a pot of water to a boil and place a steamer basket on top.

# NUTRITIONAL FACTS

- Calories: 300kcal
- Protein: 23g
- Carbohydrates: 10g
- Fat: 17g
- Fiber: 4g
- Sugar: 2g

# INSTRUCTIONS

- Add the broccoli florets, cover, and steam for about 4-5 minutes, until tender but still crisp. Remove from heat and season with salt, and optionally, red pepper flakes or additional lemon zest for extra flavor.
- Serve: Place the baked salmon fillets on plates alongside the steamed broccoli. Drizzle any leftover lemon-olive oil mixture from the baking sheet over the salmon for extra flavor.

# STUFFED BELL PEPPERS

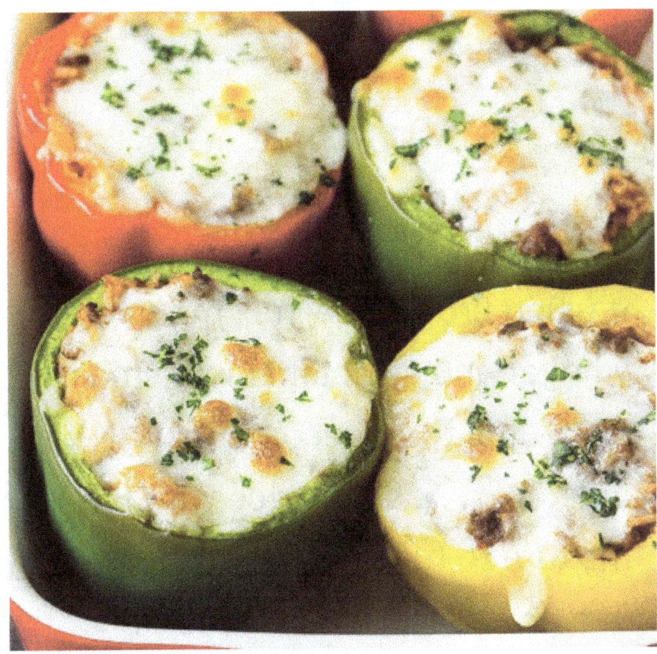

**Cook Time: 35 Mins**

**Serves: 4**

## INSTRUCTIONS

- Preheat the oven to 375°F (190°C).
- In a skillet over medium heat, cook the ground meat until it's browned. Remove excess fat.
- Add onions, carrots, and garlic to the skillet and cook until the vegetables are soft.
- Stir in the cauliflower rice and tomato sauce. Season with salt and pepper. Cook for an additional 5 minutes.
- Arrange the bell pepper halves in a baking dish. Spoon the mixture into each bell pepper half.
- Cover the dish with foil and bake for 25-30 minutes, or until the peppers are tender.
- Garnish with fresh herbs before serving.

## INGREDIENTS

- 4 large bell peppers, any color, halved and seeds removed
- 1 cup cauliflower rice
- 1/2 lb ground turkey or chicken
- 1/2 cup diced onions
- 1/2 cup diced carrots
- 2 cloves garlic, minced
- 1 cup tomato sauce (unsweetened)
- 1 teaspoon salt
- 1/2 teaspoon black pepper
- Fresh herbs (such as parsley, basil), chopped for garnish

## NUTRITIONAL FACTS

- Calories: 250kcal | Protein: 20g
- Carbohydrates: 18g | Fat: 10g

# SUSHI BOWL

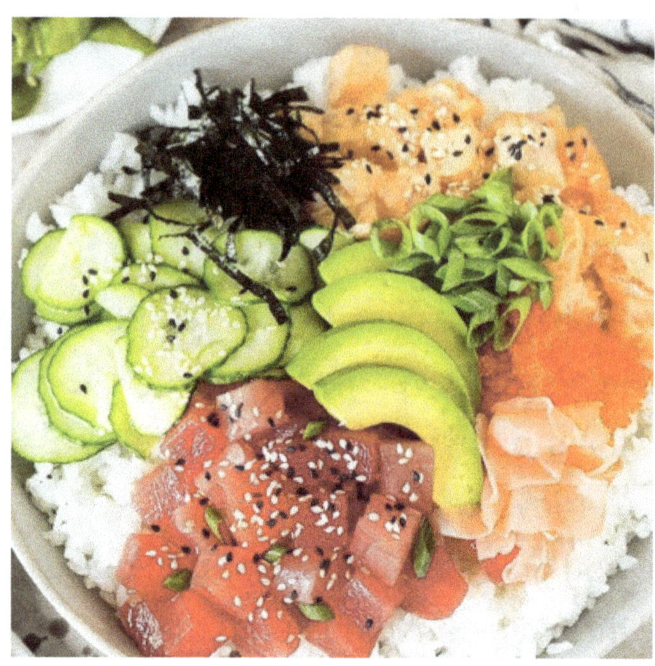

Cook Time: 15 Mins

Serves: 1

## INGREDIENTS

- 1 cup of cooked brown sushi rice or cauliflower rice (for a lower-carb option)
- 4 oz sushi-grade salmon or tuna, diced
- 1/2 avocado, sliced
- 1/2 cucumber, thinly sliced
- 1 small carrot, julienned
- 2 tablespoons of rice vinegar
- 1 teaspoon of low-calorie sweetener
- 1 tablespoon of low-sodium soy sauce or tamari
- 1 teaspoon of sesame seeds
- Seaweed sheets (nori), cut into strips

## INSTRUCTIONS

- If using brown rice, mix the rice vinegar and sweetener in a small bowl until the sweetener is dissolved. Toss the rice with the mixture to flavor it like sushi rice.
- In a bowl, start with a base of brown sushi rice or cauliflower rice.
- Arrange the diced fish, avocado slices, cucumber, and carrot on top of the rice.
- Drizzle with soy sauce or tamari and sprinkle with sesame seeds.
- Add strips of seaweed around the sides of the bowl.
- Garnish with pickled ginger, wasabi, and sriracha mayo if desired.

## NUTRITIONAL FACTS

- Calories: 600kcal | Protein: 23g
- Carbohydrates: 45g (less with cauliflower rice) | Fat: 22g

# BAKED LEMON GARLIC COD

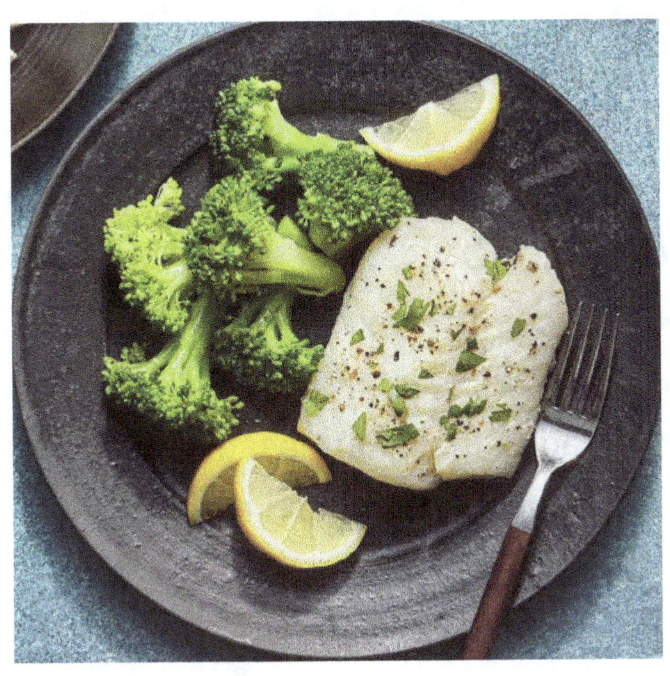

**Cook Time: 14 Mins**

**Serves: 4**

## INGREDIENTS

- 4 cod fillets (about 6 ounces each)
- 2 tablespoons olive oil
- 4 garlic cloves, minced
- Zest and juice of 1 lemon
- 1 teaspoon dried parsley (or 1 tablespoon fresh)
- 1/2 teaspoon sea salt
- 1/4 teaspoon black pepper
- Lemon slices for garnish

## INSTRUCTIONS

- Preheat the oven to 400°F (200°C).
- In a small bowl, combine olive oil, minced garlic, lemon zest, lemon juice, parsley, salt, and pepper.
- Place the cod fillets in a baking dish lined with parchment paper.
- Spoon the lemon garlic mixture over the cod fillets, ensuring they are evenly coated.
- Top each fillet with a slice of lemon.
- Bake in the preheated oven for 12-14 minutes, or until the fish easily flakes with a fork.

## NUTRITIONAL FACTS

- Calories: 190kcal
- Protein: 31g
- Carbohydrates: 2g
- Fat: 7g

# HERB-CRUSTED SALMON

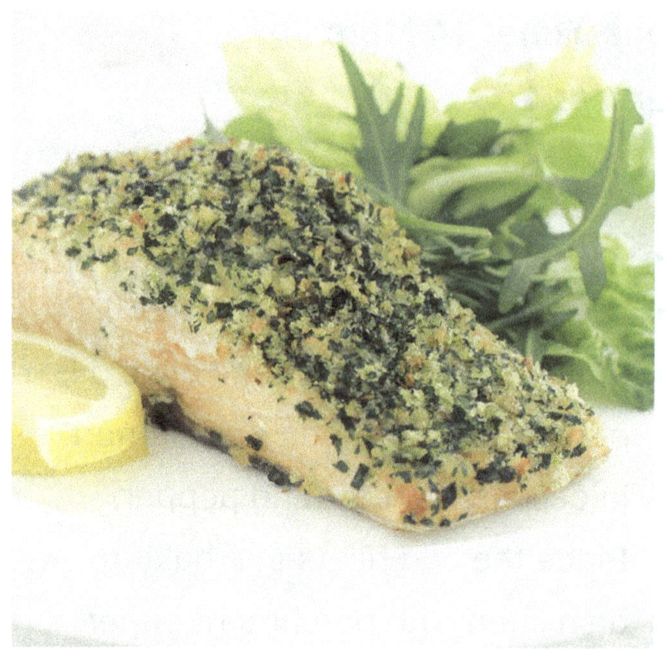

**Cook Time: 14 Mins**

**Serves: 4**

## INGREDIENTS

- 4 salmon fillets (around 6 ounces each)
- 2 tablespoons Dijon mustard
- 2 tablespoons olive oil
- 1/2 cup whole wheat panko breadcrumbs
- 1/4 cup grated Parmesan cheese
- 1/4 cup finely chopped fresh parsley
- 1 tablespoon chopped fresh dill
- 1 tablespoon chopped fresh chives
- 2 cloves garlic, minced
- Zest of 1 lemon
- Salt and pepper to taste

## INSTRUCTIONS

- Preheat the oven to 425°F (220°C).
- In a bowl, combine the panko breadcrumbs, Parmesan, parsley, dill, chives, garlic, and lemon zest. Add salt and pepper to taste.
- Lightly coat each salmon fillet with olive oil, then spread a thin layer of Dijon mustard on top.
- Press the herb and breadcrumb mixture onto the mustard-coated side of the salmon to create a crust.
- Arrange the salmon fillets on a parchment-lined baking sheet.
- Bake for 12-15 minutes, until the salmon is fully cooked and the crust is golden brown.

## NUTRITIONAL FACTS

- Calories: 190kcal
- Protein: 31g | Carbs: 9g
- Fat: 20g | Fiber: 1g

43

# ZUCCHINI NOODLES WITH PESTO

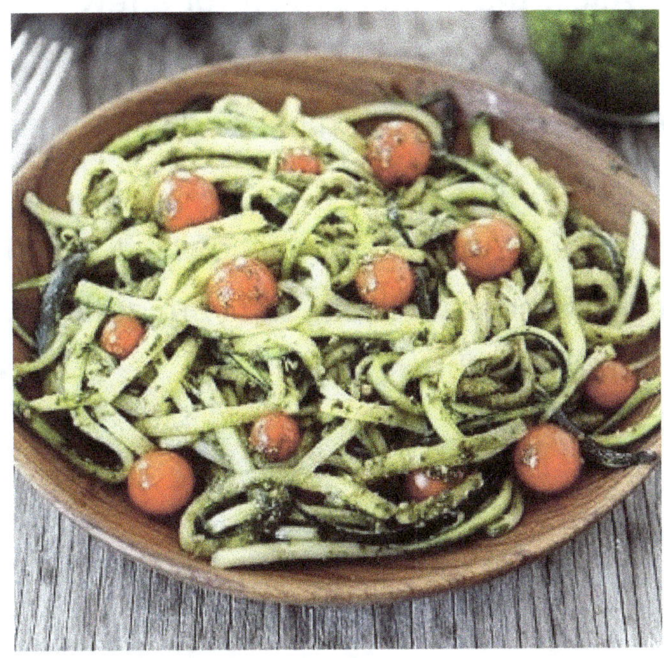

**Cook Time: 2 Mins**

**Serves: 4**

## INGREDIENTS

- 4 large zucchinis
- 2 cups fresh basil leaves
- 1/2 cup grated Parmesan cheese (use vegan Parmesan for a vegan option)
- 1/3 cup pine nuts (or sunflower seeds for a nut-free version)
- 2 garlic cloves
- 1/2 cup extra-virgin olive oil
- Salt and pepper to taste
- Lemon juice (optional)

## INSTRUCTIONS

- Place the basil leaves, Parmesan cheese, pine nuts, and garlic cloves in a food processor. Pulse until the ingredients are coarsely chopped.
- With the processor running, gradually add the olive oil until the pesto is smooth and creamy.
- Season with salt and pepper. Add a squeeze of lemon juice if you prefer a tangy flavor.
- Wash the zucchinis and cut off the ends.
- Use a spiralizer to create noodle-like strands from the zucchinis. Alternatively, you can use a vegetable peeler to make thin strips.
- In a large bowl, combine the zucchini noodles with the pesto, tossing until the noodles are evenly coated.

# NUTRITIONAL FACTS

- Calories: 250kcal
- Protein: 6g
- Total Fat: 20g
- Saturated Fat: 3g
- Carbohydrates: 10g
- Dietary Fiber: 3g
- Sugars: 5g

# INSTRUCTIONS

- Allow the mixture to sit for a few minutes to let the flavors blend.
- Dish out the zucchini noodles, garnishing with extra Parmesan cheese and fresh basil leaves.
- For a heartier meal, top with grilled chicken, shrimp, or cherry tomatoes.

# HEARTY VEGETABLE LENTIL STEW

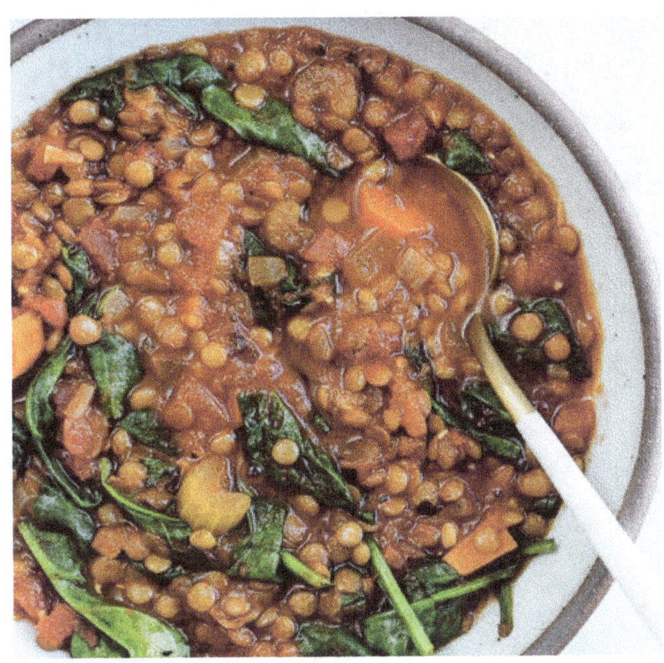

**Cook Time: 50 Mins**

**Serves: 6**

## INSTRUCTIONS

- In a large pot, heat the olive oil over medium heat.
- Sauté the diced onion and minced garlic until they become translucent.
- Add the diced carrots, celery, zucchini, and potato to the pot. Cook for about 5 minutes.
- Stir in the lentils, diced tomatoes, and vegetable broth.
- Season with ground coriander, cumin, turmeric, cinnamon, cayenne pepper (if using), salt, and pepper.
- Bring the mixture to a boil, then reduce the heat and let it simmer for approximately 40 minutes, or until the lentils are tender.
- Just before serving, garnish with fresh parsley and add a splash of lemon juice.

## INGREDIENTS

- 2 tablespoons olive oil
- 1 large onion, diced
- 2 cloves garlic, minced
- 2 carrots, peeled and diced
- 2 celery stalks, diced
- 1 zucchini, diced
- 1 potato, peeled and diced
- 1 cup French green lentils (Puy lentils)
- 1 can (14.5 oz) diced tomatoes
- 4 cups low-sodium vegetable broth
- 1 teaspoon ground coriander
- 1 teaspoon ground cumin
- 1/2 teaspoon turmeric powder

## INGREDIENTS

- 1/4 teaspoon ground cinnamon
- A pinch of cayenne pepper (optional)
- Salt and pepper to taste
- Fresh parsley, chopped
- Lemon juice

## NUTRITIONAL FACTS

- Calories: 200kcal
- Protein: 11g
- Total Fat: 3g
- Saturated Fat: 0g
- Carbohydrates: 35g
- Dietary Fiber: 15g
- Sugars: 5g

# STUFFED ACORN SQUASH

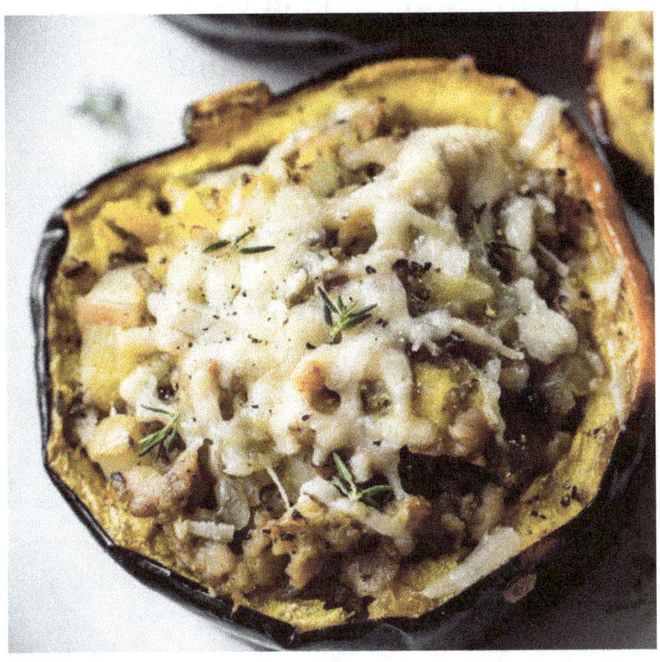

**Cook Time: 55 Mins**

**Serves: 4**

## INGREDIENTS

- 2 medium acorn squashes
- 1 tablespoon coconut oil (or avocado oil as an alternative)
- 1 pound ground pork (or compliant sausage or turkey for Whole30)
- 1 yellow onion, diced
- 3 celery stalks, chopped
- 1 Granny Smith apple, peeled and diced
- 1 teaspoon cinnamon
- 1 teaspoon sage
- 2 teaspoons thyme
- 2 teaspoons rosemary
- 1/2 teaspoon sea salt
- 2–3 tablespoons dried cranberries, without sugar or oil

## INSTRUCTIONS

- Preheat your oven to 400°F (200°C).
- Line a large baking pan with parchment paper.
- Cut the acorn squashes in half, positioning the stems downward, and remove the seeds.
- Place the squash halves skin side down on the pan, then drizzle with oil and sprinkle with cinnamon.
- Bake for 30-40 minutes, or until the squash is tender when pierced with a fork.
- While the squash is baking, brown the ground pork in a large skillet over medium heat.
- Add the diced onion, chopped celery, diced apple, cinnamon, sage, thyme, rosemary, and sea salt to the skillet. Cook until the vegetables are soft.
- Mix in the dried cranberries.

## NUTRITIONAL FACTS

- Calories: 400kcal
- Protein: 20g
- Carbohydrates: 30g
- Fat: 20g
- Fiber: 5g
- Sugar: 8g

## INSTRUCTIONS

- Once the squash is cooked, fill each half with the pork and vegetable mixture.
- Put the stuffed squashes back in the oven and broil on high until the tops are golden brown.

# ROASTED BUTTERNUT SQUASH SOUP

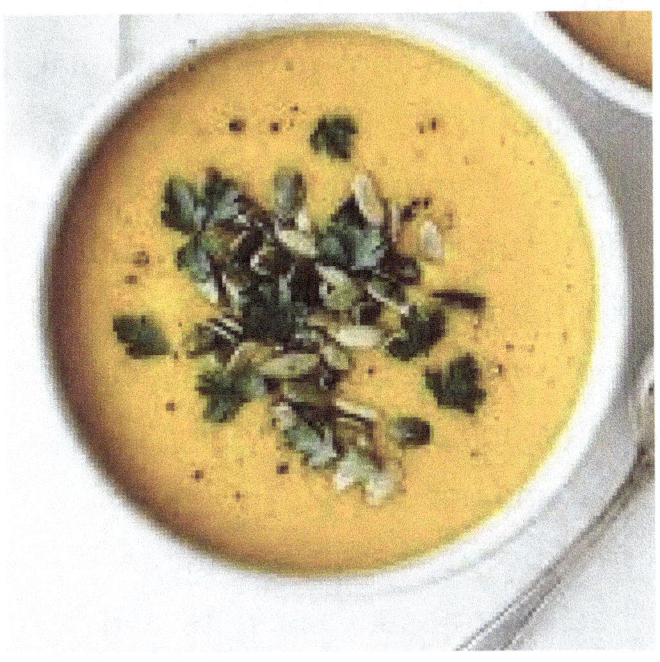

**Cook Time: 50 Mins**

**Serves: 8**

## INGREDIENTS

**For the Soup:**

- 1 large butternut squash (around 3 lbs), peeled, seeded, and cubed
- 1 yellow onion, sliced
- 4 celery stalks, chopped
- 3 garlic cloves, minced
- 1 teaspoon kosher salt
- ¾ teaspoon black pepper
- 1 tablespoon fresh sage, chopped (about 6 to 8 leaves)
- 1 cup coconut milk
- 2 to 3 cups low-sodium vegetable broth
- 4 tablespoons olive oil, divided
- Chopped chives for garnish (optional)

## INSTRUCTIONS

- Set your oven to 400°F (200°C).
- Place the cubed butternut squash on two large baking sheets.
- Drizzle each with 1½ tablespoons of olive oil and season with salt and pepper.
- Roast for 30 minutes, turning halfway through, until the squash is tender and starts to caramelize.
- While the squash roasts, heat the remaining olive oil in a large pot over medium heat.
- Add the sliced onion and cook until it caramelizes, about 20 minutes.
- Add the chopped celery and minced garlic, cooking for another 1-2 minutes.
- Pour in 2 cups of vegetable broth and bring to a simmer.
- Add the roasted squash, chopped sage, and coconut milk to the pot.

## INGREDIENTS

**For the Pesto:**

- 2 cups fresh basil leaves
- 1/2 cup grated Parmesan cheese (use vegan Parmesan for a vegan option)
- 1/3 cup pine nuts (or sunflower seeds for a nut-free option)
- 2 garlic cloves
- 1/2 cup extra-virgin olive oil
- Salt and pepper to taste

## NUTRITIONAL FACTS

- Calories: 230kcal
- Protein: 4g
- Total Fat: 18g
- Saturated Fat: 6g
- Carbohydrates: 18g
- Dietary Fiber: 5g
- Sugars: 5g

## INSTRUCTIONS

- Bring the mixture back to a simmer and cook for an additional 5 minutes.
- Use an immersion blender to puree the soup until it is smooth.
- For a thinner consistency, add more vegetable broth as needed.
- Taste and adjust seasoning with salt and pepper.
- In a food processor, blend the basil, Parmesan, pine nuts, and garlic.
- Slowly add the olive oil while blending until the pesto is smooth.
- Season with salt and pepper to taste.
- Ladle the soup into bowls, top each with a dollop of pesto, and garnish with chopped chives if desired.

# BLACK BEAN CHILI

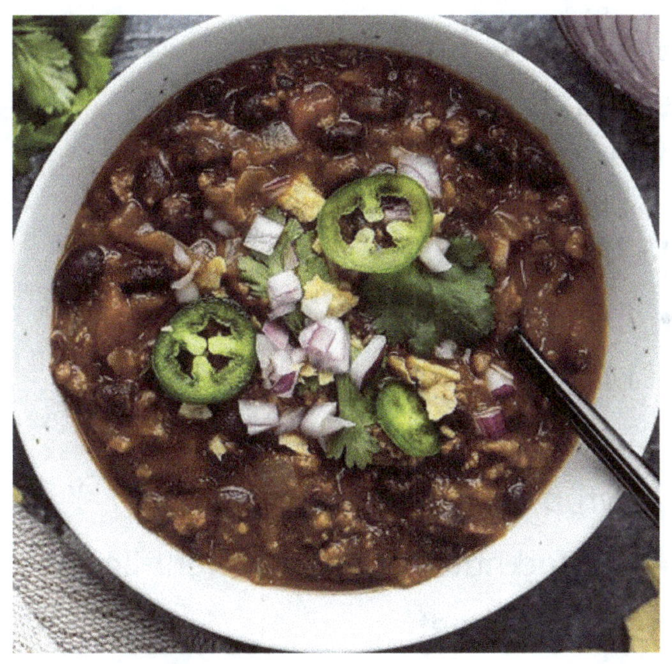

## INGREDIENTS

- 2 tablespoons olive oil
- 1 large onion, diced
- 4 garlic cloves, minced
- 2 cans (15 ounces each) black beans, undrained
- 1 can (14.5 ounces) fire-roasted diced tomatoes
- 1 jar (16 ounces) salsa verde
- 1 roasted red pepper, diced
- 1 teaspoon ground cumin
- 1/2 teaspoon chipotle chili powder (or regular chili powder)
- Salt and pepper, to taste

**Cook Time: 25 Mins**

**Serves: 6**

## INSTRUCTIONS

- Heat the olive oil in a large pot over medium heat.
- Add the diced onion and cook for about 5 minutes until it becomes translucent.
- Add the minced garlic and sauté for another minute until fragrant.
- Stir in the undrained black beans, fire-roasted diced tomatoes, salsa verde, and diced roasted red pepper.
- Season with ground cumin, chipotle chili powder, salt, and pepper.
- Bring the mixture to a boil, then reduce the heat and let it simmer for 15 minutes, stirring occasionally.

## NUTRITIONAL FACTS

- Calories: 250kcal | Protein: 15g
- Carbohydrates: 37g
- Fat: 4g | Fiber: 14g

# TURMERIC SPICED NUTS

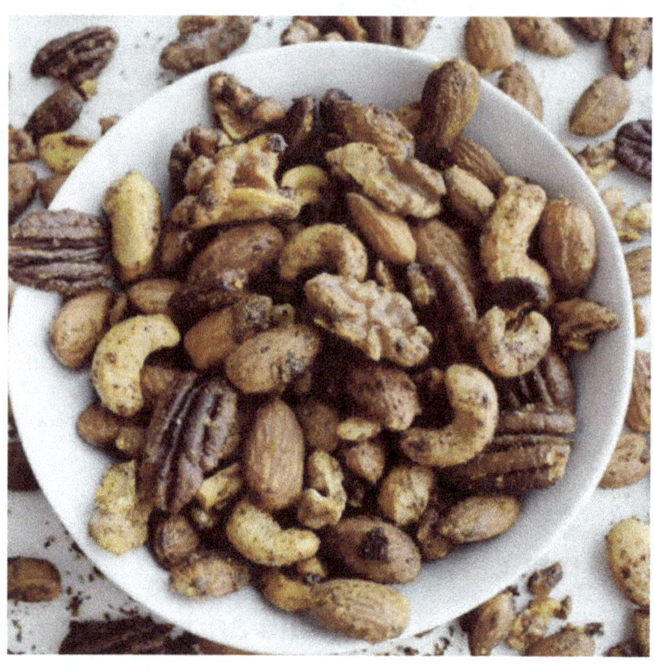

**Cook Time: 15 Mins**

**Serves: 8**

## INGREDIENTS

- 2 cups mixed nuts (almonds, cashews, walnuts, and pecans)
- 1 tablespoon olive oil
- 1 teaspoon ground turmeric
- 1/2 teaspoon ground cumin
- 1/2 teaspoon ground paprika
- 1/4 teaspoon ground black pepper
- 1/4 teaspoon cayenne pepper (optional for extra spice)
- 1/2 teaspoon sea salt
- 1 tablespoon honey or maple syrup (optional for a touch of sweetness)

## INSTRUCTIONS

- Preheat oven to 350°F (175°C).
- Mix nuts with olive oil and spices in a bowl. Add honey or maple syrup if desired.
- Spread nuts on a parchment-lined baking sheet.
- Bake for 10-15 minutes, stirring halfway through.
- Cool completely before serving or storing.

## NUTRITIONAL FACTS

- Calories; 200kcal
- Total Fat: 18g
- Carbohydrates: 7g
- Dietary Fiber: 3g
- Sugars: 2g
- Protein: 5g

# GARLIC VEGGIES WITH BAKED TEMPEH

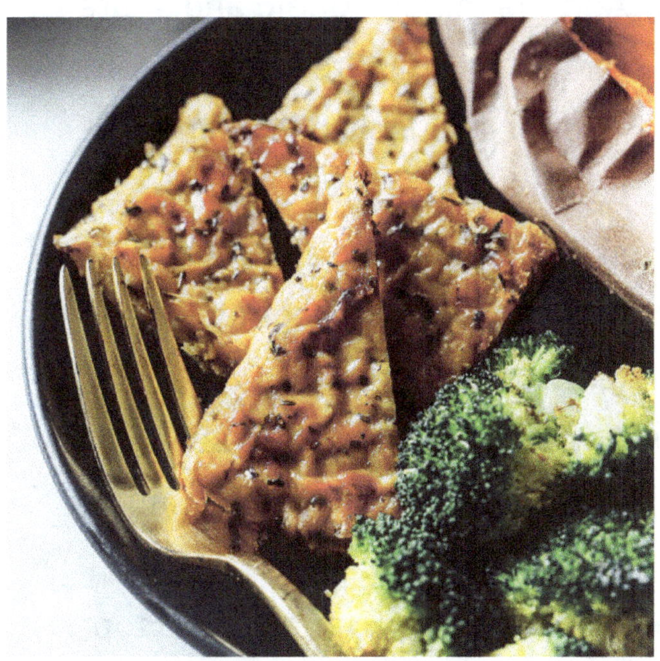

**Cook Time: 25 Mins**

**Serves: 3**

## INGREDIENTS

**For the Garlic Veggies:**

- 2 cups broccoli florets
- 1 cup sliced bell peppers (red, yellow, or green)
- 1 cup sliced carrots
- 1 cup snap peas
- 2 cloves garlic, minced
- 2 tablespoons olive oil
- 1 tablespoon soy sauce (or tamari for gluten-free)
- Salt and pepper to taste

## INSTRUCTIONS

- Preheat your oven to 375°F (190°C).
- In a bowl, mix together the soy sauce, olive oil, maple syrup, apple cider vinegar, smoked paprika, garlic powder, onion powder, salt, and pepper.
- Add the sliced tempeh to the bowl, making sure each piece is well-coated with the marinade. Let it sit for at least 10 minutes to absorb the flavors.
- Place the tempeh slices on a baking sheet lined with parchment paper. Bake for 20-25 minutes, flipping halfway through, until the tempeh is golden brown and crispy on the edges.
- While the tempeh is baking, heat 2 tablespoons of olive oil in a large skillet over medium heat.

## INGREDIENTS

**For the Baked Tempeh:**

- 1 block tempeh (8 oz), sliced into thin strips
- 2 tablespoons soy sauce (or tamari for gluten-free)
- 1 tablespoon olive oil
- 1 tablespoon maple syrup
- 1 tablespoon apple cider vinegar
- 1 teaspoon smoked paprika
- 1/2 teaspoon garlic powder
- 1/2 teaspoon onion powder
- Salt and pepper to taste

## NUTRITIONAL FACTS

- Calories: 320kcal
- Protein: 16g
- Carbohydrates: 30g
- Dietary Fiber: 6g
- Sugars: 8g
- Fat: 16g

## INSTRUCTIONS

- Add the minced garlic and sauté for about 1 minute until fragrant.
- Add the broccoli, bell peppers, carrots, and snap peas to the skillet. Stir-fry for about 5-7 minutes until the vegetables are tender but still crisp.
- Add the soy sauce and stir well to combine. Season with salt and pepper to taste.
- Plate the garlic veggies and top with the baked tempeh slices.
- Serve hot, optionally with a side of brown rice or quinoa.

# GRILLED TURKEY BREAST

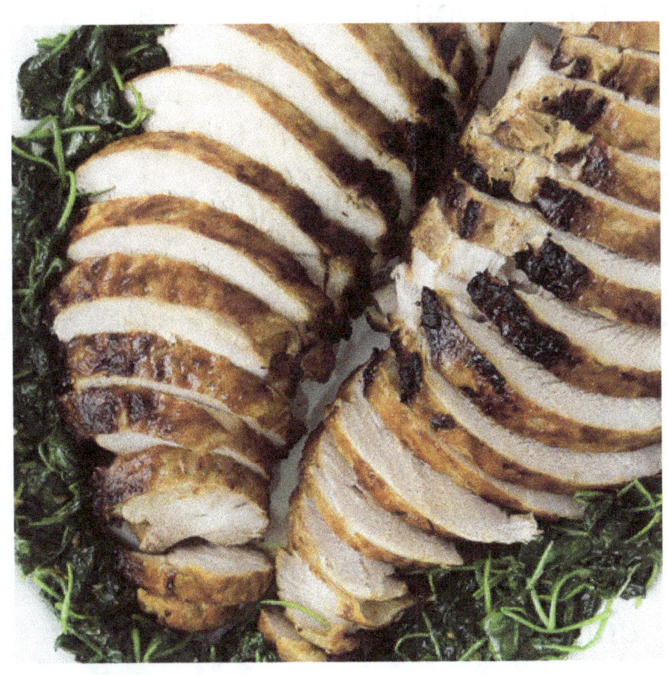

**Grill Time: 16 Mins**

**Marinate Time: 1 Hr**

**Serves: 4**

## INGREDIENTS

- 2 lbs (about 900 g) boneless, skinless turkey breast
- 2 tablespoons olive oil
- 1 tablespoon lemon juice
- 3 cloves garlic, minced
- 1 teaspoon dried thyme
- 1 teaspoon dried rosemary
- 1 teaspoon paprika
- 1 teaspoon salt
- 1/2 teaspoon black pepper

## INSTRUCTIONS

- In a small bowl, combine the olive oil, lemon juice, minced garlic, dried thyme, dried rosemary, paprika, salt, and black pepper.
- Mix well to form a marinade.
- Place the turkey breast in a large resealable plastic bag or a shallow dish.
- Pour the marinade over the turkey breast, ensuring it is evenly coated.
- Seal the bag or cover the dish and refrigerate for at least 1 hour, or overnight for best results.
- Preheat your grill to medium-high heat (around 375-400°F or 190-200°C).
- Remove the turkey breast from the marinade, allowing any excess marinade to drip off.
- Place the turkey breast on the grill.

## NUTRITIONAL FACTS

- Calories: 220kcal
- Protein: 32g
- Carbohydrates: 1g
- Fat: 9g
- Fiber: 0g
- Sugar: 0g

## INSTRUCTIONS

- Grill for about 6-8 minutes per side, or until the internal temperature reaches 165°F (74°C). Use a meat thermometer to ensure doneness.
- If the turkey breast is thick, consider slicing it horizontally into thinner pieces for more even cooking.
- Remove the turkey breast from the grill and let it rest for 5-10 minutes before slicing. This helps retain the juices and ensures a moist texture.
- Slice and serve the grilled turkey breast with your choice of sides, such as a green salad or steamed vegetables.

# CUCUMBER HUMMUS BITES

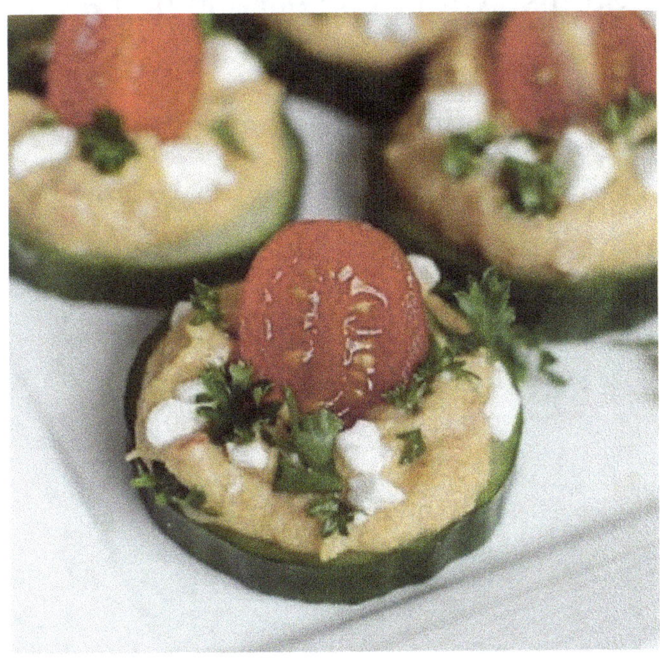

**Prep Time: 15 Mins**

**Serves: 4**

## INGREDIENTS

- 2 large cucumbers
- 1 cup hummus (store-bought or homemade)
- 1 tablespoon olive oil
- 1 teaspoon paprika (optional)
- Fresh dill, finely chopped, for garnish
- Cherry tomatoes, halved, for garnish (optional)
- Salt and pepper to taste

## INSTRUCTIONS

- Wash and dry the cucumbers.
- Cut the cucumbers into 1/2-inch thick slices.
- Using a melon baller or small spoon, scoop out a small indentation in the center of each cucumber slice, making sure not to scoop all the way through.
- If using store-bought hummus, transfer it to a bowl and stir in 1 tablespoon of olive oil until smooth.
- If making homemade hummus, blend chickpeas, tahini, lemon juice, garlic, olive oil, and spices in a food processor until smooth.
- Spoon a small amount of hummus into the indentation of each cucumber slice.
- Sprinkle a pinch of paprika on top of each hummus-filled cucumber slice if desired.

## NUTRITIONAL FACTS

- Calories: 100kcal
- Protein: 3g
- Carbohydrates: 10g
- Dietary Fiber: 3g
- Sugars: 2g
- Fat: 5g

## INSTRUCTIONS

- Garnish with fresh dill and half a cherry tomato if using.
- Lightly sprinkle the cucumber bites with salt and pepper to taste.
- Arrange the bites on a serving platter and serve immediately.

# KALE CHIPS

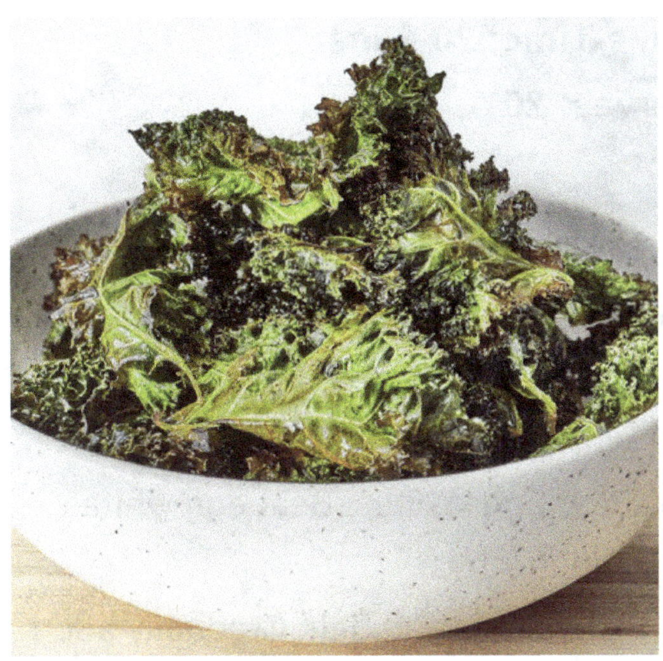

## INGREDIENTS

- 1 bunch of kale
- 1 tablespoon olive oil
- 1/2 teaspoon sea salt (optional)
- 1/2 teaspoon garlic powder (optional)
- 1/2 teaspoon smoked paprika (optional)

## NUTRITIONAL FACTS

- Calories; 200kcal
- Total Fat: 18g
- Carbohydrates: 7g
- Dietary Fiber: 3g
- Sugars: 2g
- Protein: 5g

**Cook Time: 25 Mins**

**Serves: 4**

## INSTRUCTIONS

- Preheat your oven to 300°F (150°C).
- Wash the kale thoroughly and dry it completely. Remove the stems and tough center ribs, then tear the kale leaves into bite-sized pieces.
- Place the kale pieces in a large bowl. Drizzle the olive oil over the kale and gently massage it into the leaves to ensure even coverage. If using, sprinkle the sea salt, garlic powder, and smoked paprika over the kale and toss to coat evenly.
- Spread the kale pieces out in a single layer on a baking sheet lined with parchment paper.
- Bake in the preheated oven for 20-25 minutes, until the edges are crispy but not burnt. Keep an eye on them to prevent overcooking.
- Serve immediately or store in an airtight container for up to 2 days.

# COCONUT MACAROONS

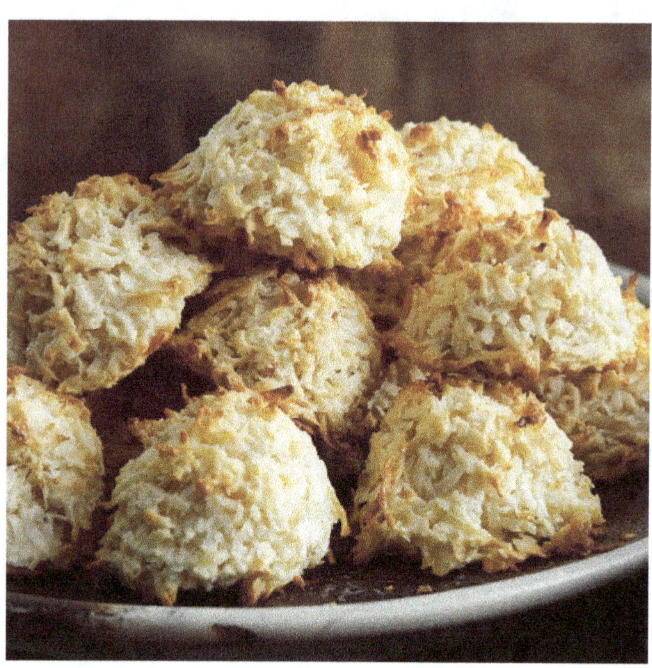

**Bake Time: 20 Mins**
**Serves: 20**

## INSTRUCTIONS

- Preheat: Preheat oven to 325°F (165°C) and line a baking sheet with parchment paper.
- Beat Egg Whites: Beat egg whites until frothy.
- Add Sugar and Salt: Gradually add coconut sugar and salt, beating until stiff peaks form.
- Fold in Vanilla: Gently fold in vanilla extract.
- Combine Dry Ingredients: Mix shredded coconut and almond flour in a bowl. Fold into the egg white mixture.
- Shape: Drop spoonfuls onto the baking sheet, spacing 1 inch apart.
- Bake: Bake for 18-20 minutes until edges are golden brown.
- Cool: Cool on the baking sheet for a few minutes, then transfer to a wire rack.

## INGREDIENTS

- 3 large egg whites
- 1/2 cup coconut sugar
- 1/4 teaspoon sea salt
- 1 teaspoon vanilla extract
- 3 cups unsweetened shredded coconut
- 1/4 cup almond flour

## NUTRITIONAL FACTS

- Calories: 75kcal
- Total Fat: 5g
- Carbohydrates: 7g
- Dietary Fiber: 2g
- Sugars: 4g
- Protein: 2g

# ROASTED CHICKPEAS

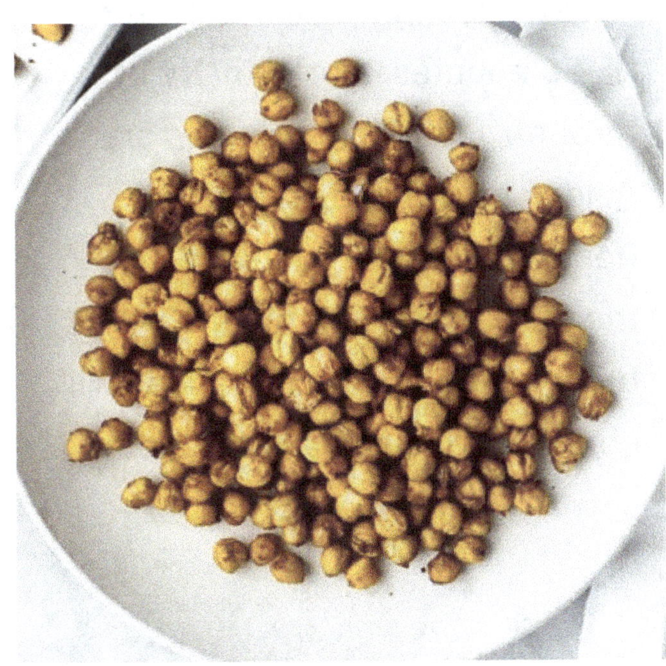

**Cook Time: 30 Mins**

**Serves: 4**

## INGREDIENTS

- 1 can (15 ounces) chickpeas, drained and rinsed
- 1 tablespoon olive oil
- 1 teaspoon ground cumin
- 1 teaspoon smoked paprika
- 1/2 teaspoon garlic powder
- 1/2 teaspoon onion powder
- 1/4 teaspoon cayenne pepper (optional)
- 1/2 teaspoon salt
- 1/4 teaspoon black pepper

## INSTRUCTIONS

- Preheat your oven to 400°F (200°C). Line a baking sheet with parchment paper or a silicone baking mat.
- Spread the drained and rinsed chickpeas on a clean kitchen towel or paper towels. Pat them dry thoroughly to ensure they roast evenly.
- In a medium-sized bowl, combine the olive oil, ground cumin, smoked paprika, garlic powder, onion powder, cayenne pepper (if using), salt, and black pepper. Mix well.
- Add the dried chickpeas to the bowl and toss until they are evenly coated with the spice mixture.
- Spread the seasoned chickpeas in a single layer on the prepared baking sheet..

## NUTRITIONAL FACTS

- Calories: 130kcal
- Protein: 5g
- Fat: 5g
- Saturated Fat: 0.5g
- Carbohydrates: 18g
- Fiber: 5g
- Sugars: 1g

## INSTRUCTIONS

- Roast in the preheated oven for 25-30 minutes, stirring halfway through, until the chickpeas are golden brown and crispy.
- Remove from the oven and let them cool for a few minutes before serving. The chickpeas will continue to crisp up as they cool

# BAKED APPLES

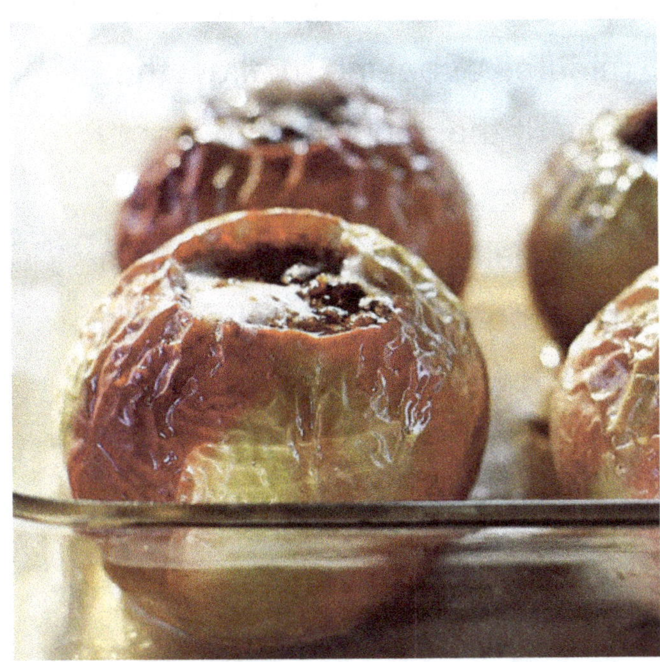

## INGREDIENTS

- 4 large apples (any baking variety like Honeycrisp or Granny Smith)
- 1/4 cup chopped nuts (walnuts, pecans, or almonds)
- 2 tablespoons honey or maple syrup
- 1 teaspoon ground cinnamon
- 1/4 teaspoon ground nutmeg
- 1 tablespoon coconut oil, melted
- 1/4 cup water

**Cook Time: 40 Mins**

**Serves: 4**

## INSTRUCTIONS

- Preheat your oven to 375°F (190°C).
- Wash the apples thoroughly and remove the cores using an apple corer or a sharp knife, leaving the bottoms intact to hold the filling.
- In a small bowl, mix together the chopped nuts, honey or maple syrup, ground cinnamon, ground nutmeg, and melted coconut oil.
- Stuff each cored apple with the nut mixture, packing it gently.
- Place the stuffed apples in a baking dish and pour the water into the bottom of the dish.
- Cover the baking dish with aluminum foil and bake in the preheated oven for 30-40 minutes, or until the apples are tender but not mushy.

## NUTRITIONAL FACTS

- Calories: 200kcal
- Total Fat: 8g
- Carbohydrates: 35g
- Dietary Fiber: 6g
- Sugars: 25g
- Protein: 2g

## INSTRUCTIONS

- Remove the foil during the last 10 minutes of baking to allow the tops of the apples to brown slightly.
- Once baked, remove the apples from the oven and let them cool for a few minutes before serving.

# DETOX GREEN SALAD

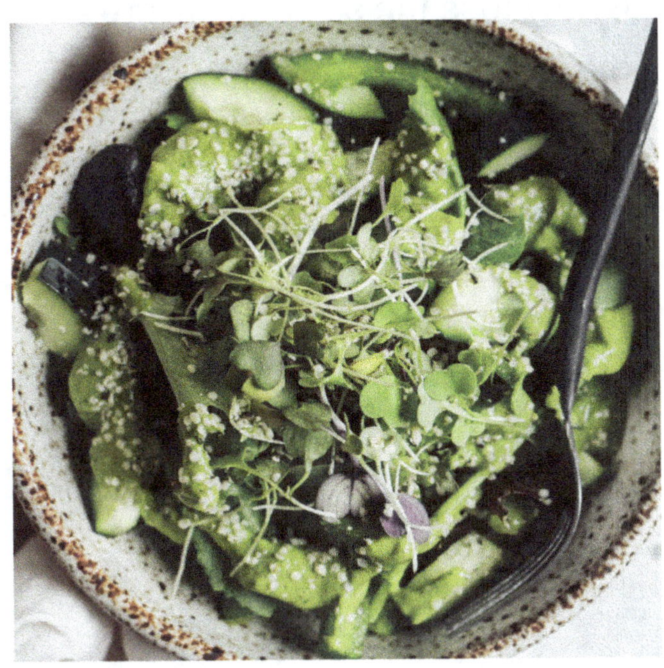

**Cook Time: 0 Mins**

**Serves: 4**

## INGREDIENTS
**For the Salad:**

- 4 cups mixed greens (spinach, kale, arugula)
- 1 cucumber, sliced
- 1 avocado, diced
- 1 green apple, thinly sliced
- 1/4 cup red onion, thinly sliced
- 1/4 cup raw sunflower seeds
- 1/4 cup fresh parsley, chopped
- 1/4 cup fresh cilantro, chopped

**For the Dressing:**

- 1/4 cup extra virgin olive oil
- 2 tablespoons apple cider vinegar
- 1 tablespoon lemon juice

## INSTRUCTIONS

- Wash and dry all the greens and vegetables thoroughly.
- Slice the cucumber, avocado, green apple, and red onion as specified.
- Chop the parsley and cilantro.
- In a small bowl or a mason jar, combine the olive oil, apple cider vinegar, lemon juice, maple syrup or honey, Dijon mustard, and minced garlic.
- Whisk or shake until well combined.
- Season with salt and pepper to taste.
- In a large salad bowl, add the mixed greens.
- Top with cucumber, avocado, green apple, red onion, sunflower seeds, parsley, and cilantro.
- Drizzle the dressing over the salad just before serving.

## INGREDIENTS

- 1 tablespoon maple syrup or honey
- 1 teaspoon Dijon mustard
- 1 garlic clove, minced
- Salt and pepper to taste

## NUTRITIONAL FACTS

- Calories: 220kcal
- Protein: 3g
- Carbohydrates: 13g
- Dietary Fiber: 6g
- Sugars: 6g
- Fat: 19g

## INSTRUCTIONS

- Gently toss the salad to ensure all the ingredients are evenly coated with the dressing.
- Serve immediately.

# SPICY THAI MANGO SALAD

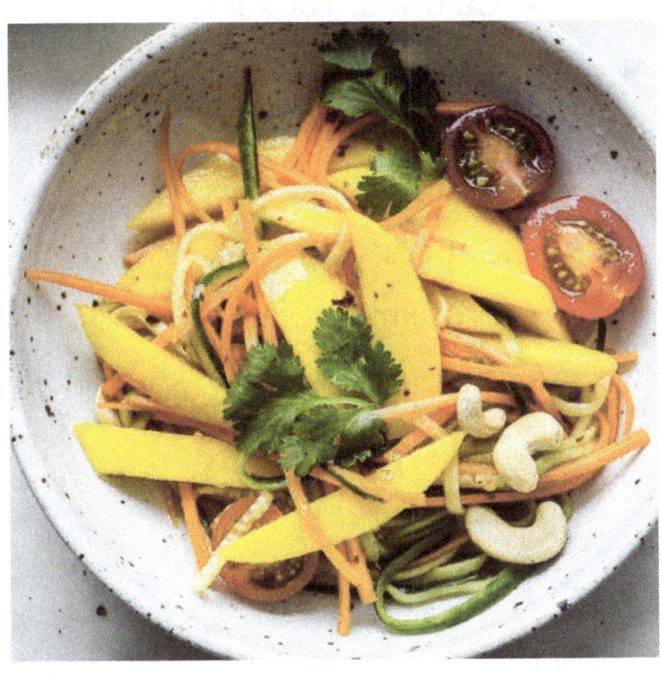

**Cook Time: 20 Mins**

**Serves: 4**

## INGREDIENTS

**For the Salad:**

- 2 ripe mangoes, peeled and thinly sliced
- 1 medium cucumber, julienned
- 1 red bell pepper, thinly sliced
- 1 cup shredded carrots
- 1/2 cup red cabbage, thinly sliced
- 1/4 cup fresh cilantro, chopped
- 1/4 cup fresh mint, chopped
- 1/4 cup fresh basil, chopped
- 1/4 cup roasted peanuts, chopped

## INSTRUCTIONS

- In a large bowl, combine the sliced mangoes, cucumber, red bell pepper, shredded carrots, and red cabbage.
- Add the chopped cilantro, mint, and basil to the bowl.
- In a small bowl, whisk together the lime juice, fish sauce (or soy sauce), rice vinegar, honey (or maple syrup), sriracha sauce, minced garlic, and sliced red chili (if using).
- Pour the dressing over the salad and toss gently to combine, ensuring all the ingredients are evenly coated.
- Sprinkle the chopped roasted peanuts on top of the salad.
- Serve immediately for the best flavor and texture.

# INGREDIENTS

**For the Dressing:**

- 2 tablespoons fresh lime juice
- 1 tablespoon fish sauce (or soy sauce for a vegan option)
- 1 tablespoon rice vinegar
- 1 tablespoon honey (or maple syrup for a vegan option)
- 1-2 teaspoons sriracha sauce (adjust to taste)
- 1 clove garlic, minced
- 1 small red chili, thinly sliced (optional for extra heat)

# NUTRITIONAL FACTS

- Calories: 180kcal
- Total Fat: 6g
- Total Carbohydrates: 31g
- Dietary Fiber: 4g
- Sugars: 23g
- Protein: 4g

# BANANA NICE CREAM

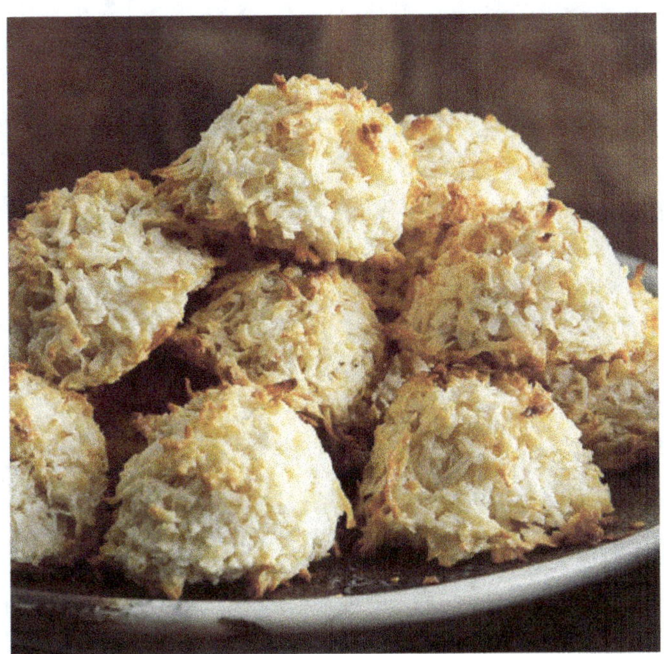

**Freezing Time: 2 Hrs**
**Serves: 4**

## INGREDIENTS

- 4 ripe bananas
- 1 teaspoon vanilla extract (optional)
- 1-2 tablespoons unsweetened almond milk or any plant-based milk (optional, for smoother texture)
- Toppings of choice (e.g., fresh berries, nuts, seeds, shredded coconut)

## NUTRITIONAL FACTS

- Calories: 105kcal
- Carbohydrates: 27g
- Protein: 1g | Fat: 0g
- Fiber: 3g | Sugars: 14g

## INSTRUCTIONS

- Peel the bananas and cut them into small chunks. Place the banana chunks in a single layer on a baking sheet lined with parchment paper. Freeze the banana chunks for at least 2 hours or until completely frozen.
- Blend the bananas until they reach a smooth, creamy consistency, similar to soft-serve ice cream. This may take a few minutes. Stop and scrape down the sides of the processor or blender as needed.
- If you prefer a creamier texture, add 1-2 tablespoons of unsweetened almond milk or any plant-based milk while blending. You can also add 1 teaspoon of vanilla extract for added flavor.
- Once the nice cream reaches your desired consistency, scoop it into bowls and serve immediately.

www.ingramcontent.com/pod-product-compliance
Lightning Source LLC
Chambersburg PA
CBHW081809250726
48653CB00010B/3859